William Standish Reed, M.D.

SURGERY
OF THE
SOUL

HEALING THE WHOLE PERSON —
SPIRIT, MIND AND BODY

Published by
CHRISTIAN MEDICAL FOUNDATION INTERNATIONAL, INC.
Tampa, Florida

Library of Congress Catalog Card Number 95-70962

ISBN 0-9648792-0-4

TO

the true physicians of the whole man (spirit, mind, and body),
beginning with Luke, and to the Great Physician, who first showed
us the Way and to Dr. Paul Tournier for his inspired thought,
which has begun to change contemporary medical practice. To
Dr. Frederick A. Coller, the great University of Michigan's professor of Surgery, to Dr. Ruth Wanstrom, professor of pathology
at Ann Arbor, the person who pointed me back to my spiritual
Christian roots. To my University - the University of Michigan.
To Ethel Tulloch Banks of the Order of St. Luke. To my beloved
wife, Kay and our children, Sue, Standish, Lyn and Rob.

A Special Note

"Surgery of the Soul" was published originally in 1959. Later on it was republished under the title, "Healing the Whole Man". Now, almost 40 years later, thanks to the loyalty, diligence and Christian commitment of Bob Stenzel, Winnie Anglin and Julie McFarland and the cooperation of Versa Press of East Peoria, Illinois, "Surgery of the Soul" re-edited and expanded comes forth once more. The chapters deal more acutely than ever with the problems encountered with healing the sick in an era of increasing turmoil and confusion. May God continue to bless this book and to bless Bob, Julie and Winnie who made the new edition come about.

WILLIAM STANDISH REED, M.D.

Contents

Introduction

With all of the technological advances of modern medical science today, it is surprising to find American medicine working toward the spiritual in its consideration of man. Four decades ago, the writings of Alexis Carrel created a furor and a storm in medical circles. Dr. Carrel, along with Dr. Howard Kelly of Johns Hopkins University and Dr. Richard Cabot of Harvard University, were pioneers of a new, vital and much-needed area in the practice of medicine and surgery, looking beyond the treatment of the physical and the mental and considering deeply the spiritual in the treatment of the whole man.

The purpose of this book is to give both physician and layman an opportunity to consider the great and relatively unexplored field of the human spirit in relationship to man's greatest enigma: consideration of himself. The religious and the spiritual in this book will be presented from the standpoint of Christianity, since the writer is a Christian and feels that, among all the religions, Christianity offers both patient and doctor the unique and limitless potential of understanding man when he is well and when he is sick. Christianity also uniquely gives man, through Christ, the power to perform both the possible and the impossible.

This book is the product of a lifetime of medical and surgical study. It is the product of a diligent search to attempt to understand man, particularly the sick man. Its research area has been not only the hospital wards and operating theaters, but also the pathology laboratory, the Church, the areas where Christians gather for prayer in the United States and Canada, as well as Europe and Eastern Europe during the communist occupation era. This endeavor has been exciting and edifying. It has proved of great benefit to me personally, as a man and as a doctor. Through this search I have found the Savior whom I see as our Healing Lord, one who not only makes me, but my patients, whole.

My prayer is that this endeavor may be useful to the physician, the nurse, the medical student, and very importantly, to the patient.

WILLIAM STANDISH REED, M.D.
Tampa, Florida

And this is the reason why the cure of many diseases is unknown to the physicians of Hellas, because they are ignorant of the whole, which ought to be studied also: for the part can never be well unless the whole is well.

Socrates

The fear of the Lord is the beginning of wisdom . . . Psalms 111:10.

1 - Beginnings

IT WAS A RATHER BLEAK, rainy night in the fall of 1939 when the bus in which I was a passenger pulled up in front of the Men's Union and let me out into what was to be the beginning of a great adventure. There was a great sense of loneliness that evening, but this was somewhat dispelled by the anticipation of entry into the university. There were many reasons why I should not have been there at all. Financial problems and physical difficulties coupled to make it seem an almost insurmountable consideration. As I recall it now, there was truly no defeatism in my attitude. I felt even then that I was in God's hands, that it was really part of God's plan for me to be walking along the rain-soaked, leaf-covered street that night with nothing but hope in my heart. No dormitory room had been provided and no one was there to greet me. It was a matter of searching out the address of an acquaintance to see if I could remain with him until I had obtained a room and hopefully a place of employment. Temporary quarters were soon obtained, and immediately I not only obtained a job which provided for my meals, but I also secured a paying position in the college symphony orchestra where I played the violin and viola. These endeavors and a job in the school of music library paid twelve dollars a month which, small though it may seem, paid for my room.

There were in the early years of student days not only earnest strivings for knowledge but also a continuing quest for the inspiration of God in life and in study. As time went on, the search for God became more dim, although He was always in my thinking. It seemed at that time that the churches I attended had very little message for me, and student activities were often only social in their consideration. As burdens of study and work became greater, activities related to the church became less and less a part of my life. In 1942, when I entered medical school, most factors which had been present when I arrived were still constant and present, except that God and the inspiration of His Holy Spirit became less consciously apparent in my life. I recall the soul-searching which I did the day I entered the anatomy laboratory, and as I began to dissect the human body, I considered what I, a human being, was actually doing in this life. I could not help reflecting upon the Psalmist's question, "What is man, that thou art mindful of him? . . . " (Psalms 8:4). As time went on, all of us became hardened to the rigorous routine of medical school and insensitive to any spiritual consideration of our studies. The human body, in its many functions, compositions and constituents, was meticulously analyzed and studied from every possible standpoint except the spiritual. The psychological aspects of disease, the physiology and anatomy of the nervous system were carefully delved into; gradually we became experts in viewing man the machine with greater and greater knowledge. No matter what the motives my former classmates may have today for being in the practice of medicine, I feel confident that all of us at that time were interested in helping human beings. Our attitude was one of compassion, with a desire to understand and help them in their suffering. There was very little spiritual emphasis placed upon any of our studies during this growth process. I do feel certain that the tremendous integrity of the medical school's very inspiring teaching staff reflected upon each and every one of us students.

Internship was not appreciably different. Here again the work load was heavy, patient contact became a matter of routine, and the emphasis of our work with the individual patient was more upon his disease than upon the person who had the disease or abnormality.

The following years of experience in the navy and in a civilian hospital found me absorbed in a desire to help people to the best of my ability as a physician. My approach was completely somatic, at best psychosomatic, giving very little thought to the spiritual aspect of patient care or the status of the patient or myself in relationship to God or to Christ.

A new world opened up to me during my training in a civilian hospital after leaving the U. S. Navy. There were the flickerings of something beyond the psychological and something beyond the somatic at that time. On one occasion, attempting to comfort the wife of a twenty-eight-year-old man who was dying of leukemia, I advised her to pray and told her that I myself would pray for her husband. This young man was one of the first patients to receive nitrogen-mustard therapy at the hospital, and as it was given, it was administered with prayer from not only the wife and the recipient, but also the young doctor who administered it. The acute myelogenous leukemia strangely became chronic, and instead of dying within days, he lived a normal life for over three years.

In another instance, a fifteen-year-old boy entered the hospital with terrible headaches and an inability to see with his right eye. Thorough studies by everyone had failed to reveal the cause of his problem. Spending much time with the patient and with his parents, I was able to determine that he had a very rare type of tumor which had spread to his brain. Here again, the only answer was to do all that we could medically and to point the family and the boy to Christ. In a fumbling way this was done, and it became a sustaining force that allowed him to die victoriously and enabled his family to accept his death.

I remember a middle-aged man who was hysterically pushing the nurse's call button in his room because he was having severe chest pain. The nurses were all busy with other patients. Although the patient was on the medical service and I on the surgical service, his need called out to me. As I dashed into his room to discover his problem, he stated that he was having tremendous pain. Not only did he state his problem, but he cursed at me because of his anger at not being served as soon as he thought he should be.

From a nurse I obtained the necessary medication; I ran to his bedside, hurriedly applying a tourniquet to his arm, attempting to find a vein in which to inject narcotic to ease his pain! The nurse was frantically trying to contact his doctor. Because of the patient's violence, his cursing and his irascibility, I could not find the vein in which to inject the medication. In the midst of this violent psychological reaction of hatred toward me and toward everyone because of our failure to please him, the man collapsed and died in my arms. I saw at that time the terrible penalty which hatred and violence can cause in an individual life.

These were but beginnings, experiences, considerations and thoughts, all pointing toward a future in which, based upon a philosophy of practice and a foundation of ethical reality, I could begin my own medical practice. I decided that the highest calling of the physician should be that of general practitioner. I thought that such a man would cover the broad spectrum of people's needs without the narrowness and the gun-barrel vision sometimes associated with one who cannot see beyond his specialty.

. . . choose you this day whom ye will serve . . . Joshua 24:15.

2 - The Choice

GENERAL PRACTICE was a most happy and enlightening experience. A small-town G.P. becomes very much a member of the
community and a close member of the families whom he treats.
He may not be admired from the standpoint of the profession in
general because his education is not as prolonged as the
specialist's, but the general practitioner must be a man of unusual abilities and insights. It has always seemed a strange paradox to me that the man in medicine who needs the greatest knowledge of all has the shortest period of training, and the man who
needs knowledge in a very narrow segment of medicine or surgery has years of training before he enters practice. It has been
my observation that the general practitioner is often the real doctor and the specialist is often a superior mechanic in a narrow
field.

When he enters practice, the general practitioner finds that
there are very subtle pressures exerted to require him to specialize, if he is going to be able to help his patients in the way he
would most desire. There was a time when most babies were
delivered by general practitioners. In many areas the general prac-

titioner now may not be allowed to deliver babies, or he is only allowed to do so under the supervision of a specialist. There was a time when much of the surgery which was performed was done by general practitioners; specialists in the large centers performed only the most complicated forms of surgery. Now, in many areas, general practitioners are not allowed to do anything but very minor surgery. These factors cause the young general practitioner to practice only long enough to decide what field of specialty he desires to enter. Then he leaves his practice to become a specialist.

Thus it was for me when I found in my general practice that many of the simple surgical conditions which confronted me day to day were successfully handled as I operated upon them. However, as specialization became more a rule of the day, I began to see that, in order to be able to do surgery at all, it was going to be necessary for me to specialize. Leaving one's practice, the families he has grown to love, the babies he has delivered, and those he has helped through victories and defeats—these are difficult things to face. However, it was with great joy that I again entered university life with all its new challenges and opportunities. The surgical training itself was a strict discipline, leaving little time for either sleep or social activity. There was the constant inspiration of the professors and others surrounding us in the various hospital departments, which made every moment exhilarating and challenging.

My chief was a man able to probe deeply into the inner depths of his patients and his residents. He neglected no aspect of his patient, including the spiritual. He exemplified the personal approach to the patient and instructed his interns and residents to comfort the patient as well as to take care of him professionally. He represented not only the surgeon as scientist but also as counselor, friend, and minister in the deepest sense of the word. Four years of training under him and his staff passed as a day, and although the opportunity was presented for me to stay on, I elected to get back to my former friends of general-practice days, to catch up the loose ends and renew friendships.

During my years of training at the university I had developed a close relationship with one of the professors of pathology. It was she who had asked me one day if I felt that Jesus Christ could heal anyone today. It was she who suggested that we study the spiritual aspect of patient care. It was she who again kindled a little fire in what had been only a flickering spark in my spiritual life. As a result of the discussions and investigation which we conducted, I left the university not only as a trained surgeon, but also a person considering more and more deeply the spiritual aspect of patient care.

As the realization deepened of how powerful the force of prayer could be in one's life and the life of his patients, I began to pray for my patients and for those in my acquaintance who were ill. I began to see that man himself is a very limited being. As he begins to see his own limitations, he looks about him, viewing with increasing sensitivity the limitations of those about him. When man contemplates God, he tends to limit Him, measuring God by the same yardstick which he uses to measure himself. He does not see God in His limitlessness, in all of His influences upon man.

In this limited context, one might believe that God sends illness upon man, perhaps as a result of his sin, perhaps as the result of his being in an environment of sin in this world. This is a difficult belief for the physician: if God does in truth send disease, the physician is fighting against God as he makes man well. If, however, disease is a result of sin and of evil primarily, the physician is in a very comforting place as he works with God as his co-laborer, striving to destroy illness and, hopefully, the sin which causes it. It was with considerations such as these, coupled with a thorough training in surgery, that I re-entered practice, vowing to incorporate to the greatest extent possible the spiritual principles which I had just begun to perceive as real and absolutely necessary. There was to come a time of growth and of struggle, as well as times of heartbreak and discouragement. One does not lightly place himself on God's road, because such a decision carries with it not only the potential of the miraculous but also the possibility of misunderstanding.

Having worked with cancer patients and patients with other diseases which medical science views as incurable, I felt strongly at the inception of surgical practice that the most neglected area of research and of thought is the spiritual. Is it possible that many illnesses have a spiritual cause? If this area of the causation of disease is true, perhaps the correction of spiritual factors can cause the healing of illnesses which by any other means would not be possible.

What was present then, as the specialty practice of surgery began, was not only the scientific consideration of man but also a deepening interest in the spiritual as well as the psychological. Man cannot be seen as a strictly surgical entity or medical consideration; he must be seen as a whole being. He cannot be visualized purely as a physical being, since true man does not exist in separate compartments. The mental cannot be isolated from the physical. This has been proved by the multiple researches and experiences in psychosomatic medicine.

We have made the error of believing that the psychological and the spiritual are one and the same. Biblically, man is divided into three parts. "And the very God of peace sanctify you wholly; and I pray God your *whole spirit and soul and body* be preserved blameless unto the coming of our Lord Jesus Christ" (1 Thessalonians 5:23, italics mine). "For the word of God *is* quick, and powerful, and sharper than any twoedged sword, piercing even to the dividing asunder of *soul and spirit*, and of the joints and marrow, and *is* a discerner of the thoughts and intents of the heart" (Hebrews 4:12). It is a mistake, then to consider soul and spirit to be one and the same; and it is also a mistake to consider the psychological synonymous with the spiritual. Throughout this book, man will be considered to be a logo-psychosomatic being: that is, spirit, soul and body—a holistic interrelated whole. Jesus asked the hopeless man at Bethesda's pool, ". . . Wilt thou be made *whole*?" (John 5:6) and said to the woman with chronic uterine bleeding, ". . . thy faith hath made thee *whole* . . . " (Mark 5:34, italics mine). Soul and mind will be considered to be one and the same. Wholeness implies complete integration in the human life of spirit, soul and body.

In the beginning, during the development of the physician, man is seen as an unending world of fascinating facts and wondrous characteristics. Gradually, material concepts of man fade to those of an even greater world comprising the unending depths of the study and the productivity of the mind. Beyond this lies the unexplored. To date only theologians have given the spirit much consideration at all, and they have been bound by limitations of dogma, creed, and denomination. Is this a realm too far removed from the physician's consideration? Or does it, like outer space and the universe, represent a challenge which he can investigate? Can such investigation obtain facts which will, in the years to come, help man not only to understand himself, but also to achieve new insights into prevention and treatment of all forms of illness?

And the Lord said to Cain, Where is Abel your brother?. . . Genesis 4:9, (AMP)

3 - *Discipline*

CURRENT SURGICAL thought is highly scientific and technical, bearing few of the earmarks of the philosophy of surgical practice which formerly characterized surgery as an art as well as a science. Before the new resident surgeon there looms the great challenge: to help suffering humanity by applying diligently the skills learned from teachers and from study. With heart-lung machines, respirators, dacron prostheses, hypotensive anesthesia, controlled respiration, controlled cardiac arrest, and many technical devices and procedures, the surgeon tends to become a supertechnician, a statistician, an operator or a research coordinator, a reader of multitudes of articles, a writer, or perhaps even more, a working machine. The demands upon the surgeon are staggering and ever increasing. Soon after becoming established in the practice of medicine, he finds himself in a dilemma. How does one do all that is required of him surgically and scientifically and still maintain his intellect, his soul, his spirit, his family, his religion, his faith? How does the surgeon, who sees on every hand the wondrous working power of God, integrate his Christian faith into his surgical practice? Is there truly a place for God in this new technical world of scientific discipline? Inevitably, also, to the young surgeon comes the question, "What is to be done now, when nothing surgically or technically can be done?"—as in the patient with carcinomatosis or multiple myeloma or a myriad of other disorders for which we still stand by, helpless to do anything curative?

There are certain moral precepts in surgery which are more religious than they are scientific. One of these is the aim of the doctor: "To cure sometimes, to relieve often, to comfort always." Another is the rule of the surgeon: If he cannot do anything to help, he must do no harm. The Oath of Hippocrates states: "In honesty and purity I will live my life and practice my art." The surgeon may differ from ordinary man by virtue of education, knowledge, ability, and affluence. He must also ask himself as any other man, when considering a possible action aimed at another human being, "If I were in his situation, how would I wish to be treated?"

"The second (commandment) *is* like unto it (the first), Thou shalt love thy neighbor as thyself" (Matthew 22:39, parentheses mine). As doctor cares for patient with skill and concern, he is being truly religious, according to the definition of James. "Pure religion and undefiled before God and the Father is this, To visit the fatherless and widows in their affliction . . ." (James 1:27). ". . .Where is Abel thy brother? . . ." (Genesis 4:9).

Surgery, although a science, must never be divorced from its true place as a deep philosophical discipline, closer to the spirit of man than the sacred ministry itself. The surgeon, perhaps even more than the internist or the psychiatrist, deals with the deep things in the lives of men. The operating room is more than a place where certain technical things are done to men to make them well or to restore function: it is a place where lives hang suspended between life and death. There the soul sleeps, the body is insensible, and the spirit hovers in communion with God. In the hands of surgeon and anesthesiologist lie not only a life, but soul and spirit capable of being influenced for good or for evil by word or thought or act.

In Judaism there occurs a question asked in the prayer of everyone, teacher or layman, "Do you know before *whom* you stand?" Could we in surgery not well afford to ask ourselves, "Do you know with Whom you operate? Do you know before Whom you stand?"

Not only is the operating theater an area to consider in the Medicine of the Person, but also the patient's room; consultation and examining rooms are important also. Here, as well, contact occurs between doctor and patient on all three levels: body, mind, and spirit. The surgeon must never consider lightly the great trust the patient bestows upon him when he places his life and his future into the surgeon's hands. Here is an act of trust which surpasses any act of surrender of one individual to another in the whole drama of life. Without the consideration of soul and spirit, surgery becomes mere technology.

Even a surgeon who considers his actions toward his patient from a purely technical viewpoint cannot escape the fact that the patient affects the doctor himself on all three levels of the doctor's being: his spirit, soul, and body. Being a doctor carries with it not only honor, rewards, applause, and position; being a doctor also places the individual physician at center target of thoughts and fears, loves, hopes, anger, disappointment and a multitude of other emotions constantly beamed at him from patients. The development of detached professional impersonality has become the new demeanor of many physicians. This frame of professional life is not a protection against the patient-doctor relationship effect, because the doctor is in the midst of a triune relationship which cannot be escaped or sidestepped. It is a part of medical and surgical practice; a doctor is involved with the patient—his spirit, his soul, and his body—whether he desires to be or not. The patient is similarly involved with the doctor; and both of us are involved with God.

When the physician sees the deeper meaning of life and of his practice, every aspect of his work takes on a wonderful new dimension. How splendid it is to save life, to restore function. How much greater--by act or word or witness--also to give meaning to that life through the Lord Jesus Christ! What would happen if the physician, whose flesh, blood, and soul are the same as his patient, should suddenly begin to see patients as eternal beings whose needs are spiritual as well as mental and physiological? No physician would deny the need to consider man as a psychosomatic entity. How can one divorce the psychosoma from the spirit? When this is done, medicine deteriorates into a mechanical science with an occasional nod toward Sigmund Freud. The physician is taught to be a doctor first, a specialist second. As a doctor he must see the total need of the whole person and treat him accordingly. This means listening to his problem, sitting down and conversing with him, and praying with him. The concept of the whole man means more than the theoretical admission of the existence of the various aspects of the human being or of God. It means being a whole doctor ministering to the total need of the whole patient.

It is my position at this point to state that the patient cannot become whole without Jesus Christ. There is no other philosophical system or religion which gives honor to the eternal spirit of man or which shows him the means of personal salvation and the way to wholeness and to life eternal that compares in any way to Christianity. We who read scientific literature to such a demanding degree should realize that great insight into the persons of our patients and ourselves can be derived through the reading and study of the Holy Bible. Jesus Christ has much to say to us, the physicians of today.

Medical ethics have become mere rules of conduct between doctors and their patients—cold, lifeless, impersonal! Jesus Christ gives to medical ethics their true place, taking into consideration the eternal spirit and man's relationship to God. Jesus' teachings are truly more a part of our medical thinking than we know. His principles are actually more the principles of medical ethics than are the tenets of Hippocrates. The ethics of medicine have more to do with interpersonal relationships than considerations such as fee splitting or ghost surgery. Such rules have become necessary because of the deterioration of medicine into a job, a means of income, a way to affluence. Materialistic medicine, emphasizing values other than honor and love of fellow man, slowly resolves into a means of maintaining self-esteem, position, income, and status. It largely ignores the Church, the Hippocratic oath, and traditional values. The Medicine of the Whole Person relates doctor and patient to Christ, who teaches man who he really is and how patient as well as physician can become whole.

Medicine as a field of scientific endeavor requires discipline in life and study. The Medicine of the Whole Person imposes an even deeper discipline upon the life and practice of the physician. Such a discipline requires that the patient's humanity never be forgotten, and that the patient's relationship to God never be violated. Such a concept of medical and surgical practice places a greater honor upon the individual patient than is usual, and requires a deeper discipline of life and of thought on the part of the doctor. Jesus Christ, the Great Physician, shows us both, doctor and patient, the way to accomplish this life-giving, creative, and redemptive relationship.

For the Word that God speaks is alive and full of power [making it active, operative, energizing, and effective]; it is sharper than any two-edged sword, penetrating to the dividing line of the breath of life (soul) and [the immortal] spirit, and of joints and marrow . . . Hebrews 4:12, (AMP)

4 - Freedom of Life

As a physician, my interpretation of this verse would be, "For the Word of God is alive and full of power and sharper than any two-edged sword (knife), cutting even to the dissection and separation of man's soul from his spirit, of his joints from his marrow."

Every man, no matter what his vocation, profession, or lot in life, must, at one time or another, answer the question Jesus put to the Pharisees, ". . . What think ye of Christ?. . . " (Matthew 22:42). This question the individual must pose to himself; it is asked far more often than is supposed. The concerns of a busy residency in a large hospital veritably keep one from thinking as deeply as he ought about what he is doing, particularly with reference to his fellow man and to his God. This was very true in my case, and perhaps Jesus' question would have gone unanswered had I not been asked the searching question by my friend and Professor of Pathology, Ruth Wanstrom, at the University of

Michigan, "Do you believe that Jesus Christ heals today?"

Confronted with this question, it is necessary to answer. To be neutral is to deny. There was no definite reason for affirming, except that deep within, I had always carried the conviction that God *is* the Author of health and wholeness; therefore, Jesus, who is the perfect reflection of God, did heal the sick when He was on earth and does heal the sick today through His disciples.

Thus affirming, I concluded, "If we believe this, why don't we study it?" Thus began a long period of exploration running concurrently with medical-surgical studies. Through this period of endeavor I was introduced to the Medicine of the Person through the writings of Paul Tournier, M.D. My encounter with Tournier and his presentation of Christ in the practice of medicine became the turning point in my life. It was he whom God used to point me toward the Bible as well as to Christ. The Bible was God's scalpel, cutting me free from materialism.

God's Word, the Holy Bible, is life itself, possessing unlimited power. It has tremendous potential and is of such a character that it has the ability to cut, to dissect and to separate even man's soul from his spirit. Ordinarily, the soul of man is considered to be the same as his spirit. Many scriptural references could be used to show that the soul of man actually is comparable not to his spirit but to his mind. The Greek word *psuche* is the same as our word psyche, used in such words as psychological and psychiatric, — pertaining to mind. Thus we see that in order to understand the statement, we must see that there is a difference between the soul and the spirit. Man's spirit doubtless exists in embryonic or atrophic form until the Holy Spirit brings it to life at the time of his conversion. It then begins to grow as it is nurtured by the Holy Spirit and the Word of God as well as by Christian living. It is this part of man which is eternal. Conversely, if the spirit of man is taken over by evil, it grows in a perverse direction as it is nurtured by the forces of evil which come upon him through the thoughts, words and deeds of the world. The Word of God has the potential of cutting between the psychological aspect of man and his spirit, thus setting free the spirit from the soul. As man progresses in intellectuality and in knowledge, he develops a tendency to subvert his spirit. God's Word presents Jesus Christ, who is able to liberate man's spirit from its incarceration by the intellect if He is but asked to do so.

In the beginning, Eve was deceived by Satan through an attack upon her intellect. Jesus Christ makes it possible to subvert the intellect, making the spirit primary. The mind of Christ becomes our potential, liberating our spirits so that we can in truth be like Him. "Let this mind be in you, which was also in Christ Jesus:" (Philippians 2:5). "For if we have been planted together in the likeness of his death, we shall be also *in the likeness* of *his* resurrection:" (Romans 6:5). Such elevation of spirit neither destroys nor diminishes man's intellectuality. Actually, such a choice expands his mental processes. To ordinary intellectual powers he has the added gifts of the Holy Spirit, including knowledge and wisdom (*see* 1 Corinthians 12:8). Intellectual knowledge does not liberate. Man is freed through the Holy Spirit revealed through God's Word.

Interesting also is the statement in Hebrews 4:12 that the Bible has the ability to cut between the joints and the marrow. As a surgeon it is difficult to understand how this could possibly be, because the marrow of the bones is not in continuity with the joints. If Paul had said "the cutting away of the cartilage from the bone" or "the bone from the marrow." it might be more understandable. Certainly there is no anatomic problem in separating of the joints from the marrow. There must be a deeper meaning here. No person would be able to walk or function without his joints. In order for a person to be healthy, it is important for him to be able to move freely and to do so he must have normal joints. The joints cannot be arthritic or frozen in order for one to have proper function and mobility. The joints thus bespeak freedom. For a person to be healthy and to have life, he must have healthy marrow. The marrow produces the cellular elements of the blood. Certain drugs act upon the marrow and cause it to be unable to produce blood elements. Certain anemias are caused by a lack of functioning marrow. Patients with anemia are weak and lifeless because of the lack of blood cells. Thus the marrow bespeaks life.

The joints of man indicate freedom, particularly freedom of motion, and the bone marrow bespeaks life. The Bible creates a means of cutting man free from the world and from the artificial aspects of the worldly life. In so doing he is completely liberated into the freedom of the Spirit. He is also given life even unto the very marrow of his bones as the life of Christ, who is Life, is infused into every area of his being. Jesus Christ, as revealed in the Bible, gives to men who will accept Him as Saviour the means of liberation and the way to life, in contrast to captivity and death which are the products of life without Him.

See, I have set before thee this day life and good, and death and evil;
Deuteronomy 30:15.

5 - *Decision*

APPLICATION of Christian principles to the practice of medicine and surgery is a difficult consideration when viewed from a practical aspect. As long as it remains on the level of the theoretical, Christianity never creates problems. Difficulties ensue when the vital principles of true Christianity are applied to life. As long as man is considered strictly a psychosomatic being and as long as the spiritual is excluded from the consideration of doctor and hospital, there are few problems. When the spiritual aspect of man is considered not just by the hospital chaplain but by the surgeon, and when application is made of the principles of Jesus Christ to the surgeon's life and practice, misunderstandings and questions may ensue.

John Watson, the Scottish clergyman, once wrote concerning the cross of Christ, "The cross is wrought in gold and hung from the neck of light-hearted beauty; it stands out in bold relief on churches that are filled with easygoing people. The cross has been taken out of Jesus' hands and smothered with flowers; it has become what He would have hated, a source of graceful ideas and agreeable emotions. When Jesus presented the cross to His disciples, He was certainly not thinking of a sentiment which can disturb no man's life nor redeem any man's soul, but of the unsightly beams which must be set up in the midst of man's pleasures and the jagged nails which must pierce his soul." The decision to believe in Jesus Christ involves the acceptance of the cross.

In the application of vital Christianity to a scientific discipline such as surgery, there are bound to be conflicts and difficulties. Many present-day surgeons would state that surgery is a scientific discipline per se, having no element beyond the scientific in any sense. However, we are dealing with human beings who cannot be viewed from strictly physiological, Freudian, or evolutionary points of view. Man remains indefinable, and the complexity of his being increases with every new facet of knowledge.

A surgeon in Canada viewed with deep despair a young adult man dying of melanoma, metastatic to his liver. The liver had become so large that it filled the entire right side of the abdomen; the patient was extremely ill, requiring frequent blood transfusions. Suddenly one day, following prayer by a group of concerned individuals, the patient began improving; the liver decreased in size and finally became normal. The patient then began a complete recovery and has been well to this day.

How can one define what happened in such a case? What is there about man on the level of the spiritual which allows him to respond in such a way to prayer? Admittedly, this does not always happen, nor is it a frequent occurrence. However, such things do occur, not only on the level of individual prayer, but at healing shrines such as Lourdes and through the ministries of certain Christian ministers. Medicine must take a closer look into these areas.

The doctor who uses chemotherapy in the all-too-often vain hope of prolonging life must give thought in other directions, including the area of Christian healing. If we are to consider ourselves open-minded and willing to experiment on the level of the pragmatic, that is, with drugs and destructive surgery, radiation therapy, and similar related fields of cancer therapy where success is limited, certain Christian investigators must think also in the direction of the Medicine of the Whole Person. Medicine must become more open in this direction, since startling healings of incurable illnesses continue to occur through the Ministry of Christian Healing.

Life itself is impossible to explain. Even on the level of simple viruses, we have become expert in the description of the biologic and chemical phenomena, but we have not been able to go beyond observation. The more minute our observations of man, the more amazed we become at the complexity and the wonder of him.

Certain ground rules have become firmly established in the realm of metabolic and physiochemical factors. No surgeon could even begin to consider the performance of major surgery on a patient without a thorough knowledge of the metabolic balance and a multitude of related factors. However, it is amazing to note that the end results of therapy in such a condition as carcinoma of the breast are little better than the results of William Halstead at the turn of the century! Perhaps it is time for the researchers to expand their horizons to include a consideration of the spiritual, not only in the treatment of the sick individual but in the prevention of physical and psychological illness. This requires something beyond launching an ordinary scientific investigation. No man can investigate these realms without first thoroughly coming to an understanding of himself and his relationship to God through Jesus Christ. One cannot approach God trusting in his own righteousness or in an attitude other than humility.

Paul's letter to the Corinthians (*see* chapter 13) can be paraphrased from the point of view of the practitioner of medicine. The paraphrase below makes one see how medicine, or any area of life, could be oriented toward a higher path.

1. Though my tongue be endued with the speech of angels with absolute completeness in all areas of man's intellectuality, and though I should speak with the inspired genius of my profession but lack the compassion of Christ, I am in reality but a hollow-sounding, chiming cymbal.

2. Though I be endowed with the deepest insight and diagnostic intuition added to a rational grasp of causes and cures of human disease; although I have superior skills in the surgical ability to excise diseased organs and tissues; although I can bind up broken bodies and minds, if I lack compassion for human suffering, I am ineffectual as a conveyor of life and preserver of wholeness.

3. Though I invest all my substance in the cause of research, even allowing my own body to be dissected in the anatomy laboratory, if I do not have divine compassion it profits me nothing.

4. The deep and sacrificial love of a doctor for his patients causes physical and emotional suffering, but the good physician's life never loses its kindness. In this deep love there is no envy,

no pride, no self-esteem.

5. In this deeper aspect of professional life there is no disorderliness; there is no seeking after the aims and objectives of self or of professional groups or societies. There is no easy provocation to anger, and evil thoughts toward one's self or others are dispelled.

6. There is no joy because of the evil or ill happening to colleagues or others, but there is great rejoicing when truth is expounded and when Jesus, who is the Truth, is lifted up. Deep love toward colleague and patient is able to bear all problems and all joys. It allows a continuing belief in the good. Not only is it accompanied by the giving forth of hope to all patients, no matter how serious their disease, but it forbids hopelessness even in the life of the doctor himself. Come what may, the life of God's love is able to endure all.

7. God's love never fails, but though there be great scientific lectures on all manner of disease phenomena and though there be all manner of intellectual pursuits, these shall eventually be no longer necessary. Inspired utterances in one's own devotional life or in the church or public meeting, even these shall eventually disappear. In the realm of professional knowledge and all of the areas of scientific advancement, present and future, in the divine scheme of things these too eventually will pass away. For now we only have a partial knowledge, and in this knowledge, we can see only a part of what is true.

8. When Jesus comes again with all of His perfection, our

partial methods will evaporate as the dew before the rising sun, for His completeness shall reveal it all.

9. Despite all professional attainments and all the knowledge which we can accumulate in this short span of our years, we are but children in our learning and in our abilities, compared with what shall be eventually revealed in us. Therefore, we must see that we speak but as children and have limited understanding in our immaturity. We think as children do, but as we achieve the maturity which is full manhood (spirit, mind - soul and body), our childish and immature areas are put away, through Jesus' own perfection working in us.

10. We get but little glimpses of the light of Christ in this present darkness, but soon, when Jesus comes, we shall see Him face-to-face and His Truth shall be revealed.

11. So in our professional lives, as we have faith in Him and as we give faith to those who are our patients and our colleagues, let us always be conveyors of hope, abounding in hope and abounding in the sacrificial Love of Jesus. Of these three values, let us remember that above all there is the deep and continuing love of God Himself, which dwells in these vessels of clay, our bodies, in which His Holy Spirit abides—if we but will Him so to do.

One of the great disappointments in the sensitive young surgeon is the gradual shattering of many of his illusions and dreams relative to the practice of surgery. He may find it difficult to be a conveyor of hope, and the tendency toward cold professionalism makes it difficult to express love to his patient. It is almost as if he is afraid to get too close to his patient, lest affection and caring diminish his professional acumen.

He sees in his professors and those who teach him a demeanor toward patients which is not always caring. The operation or the treatment may be carried out with spectacular efficiency, but the person who is being treated is somehow lost. Diagnostic evaluations may be carried out to the point of exhaustion of the patient in the, at times, vain attempt to determine a diagnosis.

Love, hope, peacefulness and joy can be part of the practice of medicine and surgery, but as medicine unfolds in our century, we find that these wonderful fields are becoming destitute of the higher virtues. We have sacrificed everything to the god of expediency and efficiency, and too often we have forgotten that the reason we went into the profession of medicine was to take care of poor sick and dying people. We did not enter the field in order to accumulate wealth or in order to amass power unto ourselves.

The demeanor of our society and the orientation of our professional groups tend toward the mad search for fame and position, and in the scramble and rush, we tend to forget the patient and our families, which to me is a great tragedy. In a trip in 1975 to Poland, where I spoke to physicians and nurses, and in a subsequent trip to Czechoslovakia, where again I met with doctors and their families, I found that American materialism can be a greater detriment to the physician and to the nurse than atheistic communism. Materialism is an opiate which destroys character and erodes human values without even the cognizance that those values are being destroyed. Atheistic communism, by contrast, is an absolute fact which must be viewed in a concrete fashion day by day, and is not something which destroys the spirit and soul of the individual without being discerned, as is often true with materialism.

Thus we must rediscover the spiritual values of Whole-Person Medicine and must orient medical and nursing lives and patient care toward the Lord Jesus Christ and the power of His Holy Spirit. This must be done urgently and immediately, without further delay. Because of the problems with medical practice as it exists at the moment, various avenues are being suggested which would bring about radical changes in patient care and in the performance of medical, psychiatric, and surgical skills. The nationalization of medicine would certainly create a massive upheaval in the entire area of patient care. It is absolutely true that there is a great need for change, but the change should not be in the direction of nationalization or socialization of medicine, by whatever term it is called.

Another avenue of change of medical practice is that which has been called holistic medicine. The primary concept of holistic medicine is that of the patient being the primary entity to be considered in medical, surgical, and psychiatric care. One of the great keystones of holistic medical thought is that diseases should be prevented, foreseen, and eliminated before they occur. Many patients have physical predispositions toward certain illnesses through their heredity, their environment, and their basic physical structure. Also, human beings possess basic and differing psychological potentialities. The individual patient should know what these potentials for bad and good are and how the unfolding of life as it affects these potentials will make the development of certain disease states possible.

The aim of Whole-Person Medicine in the future should be to prevent illness, not only through public-health means such as immunization and the correction of environmental health hazards, but each person should be evaluated on the basis of his total logo-psychosomatic predisposition model for his personal life. Counselors then would examine such patients, in order to assist them in the prevention of disease. Through a much more thorough study than is now usually given to patients, counselors could determine advice patterns for the individual person, including spiritual advice, so that the person may aim toward a disease-free life and eventual death without disease.

Present medical methods have been devoted almost exclusively to the treatment of disease states and the treatment of iatrogenic (doctor-and-medication-produced) disorders. The performance of coronary bypass operations for the treatment of coronary atherosclerosis is a case in point. The bypassing of an obstructed coronary artery through the use of a vein graft is only temporizing the problem. The atherosclerosis of the vessel and of the entire circulatory system remains untreated. Coronary bypass surgery, and most arterial bypass surgery, is simply stopgap treatment prior to the eventual development of further circulatory catastrophes. Relatively little is being done in medicine concerning the prevention of atherosclerosis, strokes, cardiovascular disease, gallstones and a multitude of stress conditions and degenerative processes. We have contented ourselves with the treatment of the failing heart, the treatment of the developed cancer of the breast, the oncologic treatment of metastatic disease, and the treatment of the degenerating and deteriorating human in general.

How different this is from Christ's statement that He came

that we might have life and that we might have it more abundantly (*see* John 10:10). It is my feeling that holistic medicine has pointed out to physicians that diet, environment, exercise, and the cataloging of basic predisposition to various disease processes are important. My personal disagreement with holistic medicine lies in its tendency to incorporate psychic and spiritualistic meditative endeavors into its framework. As a Christian, I have to believe that God's Word is correct when it states that the carnal mind eventuates in death. Medicine today is having great difficulties because it has concentrated its entire endeavor in the area of the psychosomatic (the carnal mind). It is thus apparent why our hospitals cannot be made large enough, why our mental hospitals are too small, and why our prisons are full. Psychic healing and holistic medicine continue to be in the area of the psychosomatic, ignoring true Christian spirituality.

In Romans 8:6, the Bible says that to be spiritually minded is life and peace. In other words, what we must begin to do is to consider man as a whole person—spirit, soul and body—and begin to treat the person spiritually. We must begin to see that when man is born again (born of the Spirit), his spiritual life must be his primary consideration, and his life must be spiritual. If his life is not spiritual and is simply psychosomatic, he then is involved in a death system which will eventuate in disease and death if it is allowed to go unmodified. The human being was created in the image of God. He must be spirit, soul, and body, and he can only become this way through being born of the Spirit. This does not mean born of the psyche, which the psychic healers and the spiritualists would have us believe. The meditative cults, including Transcendental Meditation, are simply psychic endeavors which are not part of the logos. We must begin to know what becoming spiritual is, and that man can only become spiritual through acceptance of Jesus Christ as his personal Saviour and Lord and by being filled with and controlled by His Holy Spirit.

Whole-Person Medicine can only be practiced by born-again, Spirit-filled physicians and nurses. Their endeavor in patient treatment must be to see that patients are led to a saving knowledge of Jesus Christ. When patients begin to live and move and have their being in Jesus, and are empowered by the Holy Spirit, they have within their being the seeds of wholeness and the endowments of the Holy Spirit termed gifts of healing (*see* 1 Corinthians 12:9). This change in medical and nursing practice allows the true discovery of the identity of the patient. The doctor and nurse will also determine their true identity.

It is becoming increasingly apparent that present modalities of treatment are not producing greater quality of life, nor longevity. On a world-wide scale, there is no relationship of increasing medical costs to remaining life expectancy. Something is missing. There is a lack, a deficiency, and the problem appears to increase the more we pour money and endeavor into the psychosomatic system. Modern man is losing life and its quality, and our national medical endeavors only increase the destructive process (catabolism). Huge hospitals and psychiatric institutions filled to capacity are signs of our failure. Man cannot be treated successfully through psychosomatic means. The lower animals are psychosomatic, so veterinary medicine understandably is oriented only to the psychosoma. Man is spirit, mind, and body, and can only successfully be understood and treated on the basis of his triune nature, spirit, mind and body.

The laws of God are spiritual, and must be obeyed if man is

to be whole. Let us consider God's laws: (Deuteronomy 5:6-21):

1. I am the Lord they God...Thou shalt have none other gods before me.

2. Thou shalt not make thee any graven image, or any likeness of any thing that is in heaven above, or that is in the earth beneath, or that is in the waters beneath the earth: Thou shalt not bow down thyself unto them, nor serve them: for I the Lord thy God am a jealous God, visiting the iniquity of the fathers upon the children unto the third and fourth generation of them that hate me, And showing mercy unto thousands of them that love me and keep my commandments.

3. Thou shalt not take the name of the Lord thy God in vain: for the Lord will not hold him guiltless that taketh his name in vain.

4. Keep the sabbath day . . . Six days thou shalt labour, and do all thy work: But the seventh day is the sabbath of the Lord thy God: . . .

5. Honour thy father and thy mother, . . . that thy days may be prolonged . . . in the land which the Lord thy God giveth thee.

6. Thou shalt not kill.

7. Neither shalt thou commit adultery.

8. Neither shalt thou steal.

9. Neither shalt thou bear false witness against thy neighbour.

10. Neither shalt thou desire thy neighbour's wife, neither shalt though covet thy neighbour's house, . . . or any thing that is thy neighbour's.

In summarizing the law, Jesus said, ". . . Thou shalt love the Lord thy God with all thy heart, and with all thy soul, and with all thy mind. This is the first and great commandment. And the second is like unto it, Thou shalt love thy neighbour as thyself. On these two commandments hang all the law and the prophets" (Matthew 22:37-40).

The life of man has gradually eliminated the laws of God in this century. In medicine, there has been the insidious replacement of God with all manner of false gods and representations of God, which physician and patient daily bow down to and worship. God's name is frequently taken in vain by people in general. Everyone works and plays seven days a week. Parents are rarely honored, and the family unit is so decimated that children, at times, do not know who their parents actually are. Murder in our century is commonplace through war, violence, abortion, and scientific experimentation. Adultery and sexual deviation are rarely considered sinful or immoral in world society. With increasing crime throughout the world, stealing is occurring on every hand. Bearing false witness and coveting are common. Love of God with all of one's heart is rarely seen, and love of neighbor as self is virtually unheard of. How can psychotherapy, holistic healing, antibiotics, heart transplantation, and the nationalization of health care hope to change these realities?

Man is ill because he is warped and unconceived in spirit. His spiritual potential is unthought of and unrealized. He has thought that his mental energies were of spirit as well as mind, and he began to know himself and his fellowman only on the basis of mind and body. This has created the fantastic problem of modern man—dying in the midst of all of his therapeutic triumphs. Only spiritual rebirth will give life and healing.

Jesus said unto her, I am the resurrection, and the life: he that believeth in me, though he were dead, yet shall he live: John 11:25.

6 - Cancer I

THE PATIENT was a young woman, a piano teacher in her home community, who had noticed the small nodule in her breast. Since she was a believer in the Gospel of Jesus Christ, she and her friends agreed that she should pray about her abnormality and seek medical help later. Such was her mode of care. She ignored her problem and went along without concern. Within two months, she saw a physician on another matter and the mass in the breast was discovered. The physician advised her to have immediate surgery. She declined.

Many months went by, during which time the mass grew to involve the entire breast. It became inflammatory and the lymph nodes began to enlarge in the axilla. Shortly thereafter she began to have small hemorrhages from the breast. This was very debilitating. Eventually, a fellow townsman prevailed upon her to seek medical advice. An ambulance carried her across the state to receive surgical help.

When the patient arrived, multiple transfusions were necessary before it was possible to even evaluate her condition. Examination revealed an advanced cancer of the breast. In order to control the bleeding it was necessary to take her to the operating room and to remove the breast.

The patient did well following her surgery for a time, but eventually developed recurrences in the skin and in the lungs. After many months of distress, during which her only solace was prayer and her deep belief in the Lord Jesus Christ, the patient died.

The reason for detailing this patient's history is simply to indicate that it is not a manifestation of faith for a person to ignore obvious surgical indications because he feels that he is trusting God by not going to a doctor. The first thing for a patient to do whenever he has a physical abnormality of any sort is to pray and perhaps to ask the Christian community to pray for him. He then should seek his physician and follow whatever advice that physician gives. In the instance quoted above, the patient should have sought help from her physician immediately and should have had surgery as well as prayer. Had she done this, she no doubt could have been well today. Neglect is not faith. Admittedly, we do not have in medicine or surgery today the answer to the cancer problem. However, this does not mean that we should not take advantage of the knowledge that we do have. We are able to give the patient considerably more help if he is operated upon, than he would have if he neglects himself. The sooner one gets medical help or surgical help when he has cancer, the more chance he has of surviving this illness, which is so common today.

Not long ago a woman who had cancer of the breast wrote to me. Her letter indicates the proper approach although with delay, and is a most interesting example of the way in which Jesus heals the person who seeks medical advice and yet gets into difficulty.

.

"Dear Dr. Reed,

Last March, our sixth baby was born—on Easter morning. She was a beautiful girl. (My husband and I felt very blessed of the Lord for our family—now we had five girls, one boy,—all of them healthy and perfect. I had had good health, no complications, natural childbirth, and had been able to nurse each one.) It was a little upsetting to discover a mass in one breast, and while in the hospital, my Gyn man called in a surgeon. He advised a biopsy right away, but after consideration and seeing how disappointed I was at the prospect of stopping nursing, he felt reasonably sure it was a plugged gland. For the next eight months, it neither enlarged nor became sensitive—the surgeon checked it regularly. After I finished nursing, it did not go away, so he recommended minor surgery—probably a cyst.

I entered the hospital. After surgery, I woke up with two thoughts: there had been a lapse of time, and never had I known so much pain. Then my husband told me—yes, it was seven hours later, there had been radical breast removal, but the surgeon was very reassuring. It had been a plugged gland after all, but sensing something, he had discovered a pea-sized malignant tumor, in no way connected with the original problem, and was forced to do a mastectomy. He was certain he had removed it all.

It was interesting that I had a memory of great pain, but it was not the pain I was having at the present time. I was still under sedation. My recovery was rapid—returned home in ten days and in a month had almost full use of my arm. But deep inside I was very troubled. I remember just before Christmas I rode along in the car as the rest of the family went on the traditional hike at the tree farm to pick out our Christmas tree. As I watched them go, I choked back the tears and tried desperately to repress the idea that this was the last year with my family—I had better take each view in completely. Many nights I would wake up knowing that I had had a very disturbing nightmare, but never being able to recall what it was about.

The doctor had advised a hysterectomy as preventive medicine, so in January I had a pan-hysterectomy. Recovery again was very rapid, lab reports had all been negative, and truly we were rejoicing. But the nightmares continued and the last one I remembered vividly. I dreamed while my husband and I were sleeping that a sinister figure, dressed in white, with a cloth wrapped around his head, entered our room, came to the head of the bed and started talking to me. I knew I should tell Bob that this evil man was here. I dreamed I was shaking Bob to wake up, was trying to tell him, but could make only guttural sounds. Actually this *was* happening. Bob woke up, heard the grunts I was making. I could hear him talking to me and saying to wake up, but I couldn't respond. It seemed like a long time, but was only moments until I awoke and could tell him of the nightmare.

Four week's after the hysterectomy, I returned for an examination: everything had gone so well, I asked the doctor how he felt about recurrence and was stunned as I heard the words coming out, "Medically we offer you no hope. Metastasis has taken place...cancer in one ovary...perhaps you'll have as long as two years." This was on a Wednesday afternoon.

Thursday morning I called a friend and asked her to pray for us. I had really been shattered inside. She said that she and her husband had been trying to contact my husband, for they heard via the grapevine that the surgeon during the radical had said this was serious, and he'd give me a year to live. That shattered me more to think he had not told me the truth. Actually, eighteen nodes had been removed, many of them involved.

Friday I called my doctor on the phone, for I remembered they had taken a series of X-ray pictures in the hospital. Had they shown anything further? "Yes, it was also in the lower spine."

That was the lowest night of my life. After many tears, deep soul-searching, and review of our lives together, Bob and I came to several conclusions. We were still young—thirty-five—and our children were still young--the oldest eleven. We had had a very deep and meaningful relationship as husband and wife, and although we really didn't want all this to end this way, we still were willing to have the Lord's will in our lives. And even if we didn't understand all this, in faith we believed our total commitment to Christ included even this.

Saturday the doctor called and said there was a disagreement on the diagnosis of the X-ray; they did not now see it in the lower spine. Good news, yes, but I have to admit I was so shattered emotionally that I was very nauseated and had lost weight rapidly those three days.

We asked if our pastor and elders would come and pray for us. On Sunday they came, and while this has not been a practice in our church, they anointed me with oil, had laying on of hands, and a very meaningful and precious time in prayer for healing. My nausea went away and has never returned!

Along with the battle of being willing to give total commitment came the small beginning of faith to be healed. As an encouragement, I had asked the Lord to heal rapidly three dime-size spots on the large skin graft that had not changed for nine weeks. By the next morning they were beginning to dry up and in one and a half weeks were completely healed! This, plus the prayer by our pastor and elders, helped me much during the next two weeks. It seems like a real spiritual battle to resist fear and discouragement and hang on to faith to believe for healing. It was as real as Satan confronting me and speaking. "You think you are healed? Why should you be healed when people are dying from cancer every day? What about this pain in your back?" And then I would get an overwhelming pain in my back. This would happen over and over and the only way to combat it would be to pray, "Lord, I know I don't deserve to be healed, but You have been giving me faith to believe for healing. Now, I don't know what this pain is, but I just give it to You to deal with. Anything of fear or depression is not from You—You give peace and joy!" I cannot even begin to evaluate the help from the prayers of our Christian friends at this time.

After two weeks of this, in the middle of a day, a sense of someone saying."Now don't concentrate on so much of the physical, for the heat of the battle is over." swept over me. It was not a rebuke-more a guiding thing. And it was over!

A week or so later another thing, very unexpected, strange, but very real, happened. I know God deals differently with people. We are all different and individuals. I can't explain it. I just know it happened to me. I was lying down resting one afternoon, dully awake, when I was impressed with a strong picture in my mind. A line, broken in the middle, a dark-black, ugly mass boiling up and spilling out at the break, and the word CANCER above. I had never experienced anything like this and thought it was just my imagination—maybe I should just think of something else. But it wouldn't go away. So I looked at it clearly, and it changed then to an unbroken line with the words beneath, AS IF IT HAD

NEVER BEEN.

I particularly noticed that I couldn't see where the break had been--no scar to show me. I jumped off the bed, overwhelmed with the closeness, the love, and the mercy of God. I have to believe this was a promise of healing. The following week, the surgeon said this has been scirrhous cancer—it forms scar tissue. But there had been no scar in this picture! Each morning I wake up feeling excellent. It is a miracle that the Lord has given peace and you to me. I do not dread each examination. I rather look forward to it. I know this is too soon to say medically that healing has taken place. But I have to believe by faith that it has. If I waver in this I am being faithless. Each day, Psalm 103:1 is precious, ". . . and all that is within me, . . . " every cell of my body must praise Him: even undisciplined cancer cells must come under His discipline. And I can just thank the Lord and praise Him for allowing me to go through this experience! Even my neighbors realize there is a new intensity in my life. I can sing while mowing the lawn, hanging out diapers, and pulling weeds!

I wonder if the subconscious mind registered the doctor's words during the first surgery that he thought perhaps there would be a year to live? Then the nightmares were an expression of trying to communicate and tell my husband. For in spite of good reports at first from the doctor, I felt the hopelessness of the case. Can this be possible?

Two instances of cancer of the breast have been noted in this chapter. In the first case the patient decided to rely strictly upon faith that she would be healed. Much valuable time was lost and despite the fact that surgical methods were finally resorted to, the patient succumbed to her illness. This is not to say that had she sought surgical attention immediately the outcome would have been different. However, with the methods which we have available today, the only chance for the patient with cancer of the breast, as far as science is concerned, is to get to the doctor as soon as any mass is found in the breast and not to procrastinate.

Those individuals who work either within the church or outside the church in the realm of the Healing Ministry should be extremely cautious in their advice to cancer patients. They should not advise against seeking early medical and surgical attention for cancerous disease. I believe implicitly in the Healing Ministry of the Church of Jesus Christ. However, I believe that this ministry should be used in conjunction with the best medical and surgical methods—not as a substitute for scientific methods. It is my belief that the answer to the prayer of the cancer sufferers often is the scalpel of the well-trained surgeon and those who work along with him, aiming toward the total ablation of the cancerous growth.

The second patient whose letter is quoted sought medical attention early, but delay occurred as a result of a mistaken diagnosis. When surgical intervention was attempted the cancer had already spread beyond the confines of the surgical operation. The surgeon, as many surgeons are wont to do, decided to lie to his patient and tell her that the cancer had been removed, despite the fact he had stated something different at the time of the operation. He failed to realize that his statements in the operating room were made in the presence of his patient, who registered them in her subconscious mind just as surely as if she had been awake. There then followed the series of events which she describes. Finally she sought the help of the Healing Church, and miraculously she experienced first healing of her subconscious mind and her psychological problem, which then was followed by physical healing.

What can be the differences in these two patients? Both believed in the healing virtue of Jesus Christ in His Church today. Both sought the help of the Healing Church. In both instances there was procrastination—one because the patient decided to wait of her own volition, and the other because of the reassurance of an erroneous diagnosis.

There are doubtless many factors in both cases we know nothing about, but there is one which occurs to me, since I have seen more instances of the first type of patient than I like to think about. I do not believe that it is a manifestation of faith to neglect to seek help when it is available. Many people in this kind of situation substitute fear for faith. Actually, what they do is develop a morbid fear of their illness which paralyzes them from doing anything of a constructive nature with reference to their illness. They obtain some solace and some comfort from the healing ministry of the Church, but their fear remains, and their cancer, with all of its roots in the subconscious mind, continues to be present. Fear is perhaps the greatest ally of cancer and can only be removed from the person through an act of the will to do something about his illness and through the intervention of God in the total person of the individual—spirit, soul, and body. The Ministry of Healing should never be conducted apart from the doctor and the nurse, who, along with an enlightened clergy, should be the agencies of the healing love of Jesus Christ toward cancer sufferers. This is admittedly an ideal which is rarely present in an era of scientific medicine which has ignored the spiritual and been blind to the Healing Ministry.

The second case illustrates the profound need of the enlightened physician for the Gospel of healing in the medical profession today. Our lack of a spiritual approach produces a callousness and a cold impersonality toward our desperate patients. Many seek help in the terminal states of illness from the fringe areas of medicine which can promise nothing but an even more heartless using of the desperate patient and his family.

The course of the medically or surgically hopeless case is of great concern to all thinking physicians who are faced with the problem of cancer. Desperate attempts are often made by the patient or his family to achieve a cure through the use of fringe-type cancer treatments which are questionable or of no value. There is a growing number of people beginning to realize that their place is at the doctor's side in the effort to rid cancer from our lives. Some enlightened churches are holding healing services where the patient can come for prayer and unction. The Healing Church is a new phenomenon on the American scene; it is in this area that the physician as well as the patient sees an arm of support which has rarely been present before. It is to be sincerely hoped that through prayer and through the confidence which comes to the patient as a result of being surrounded by love, care and concern by a believing fellowship, miraculous things can occur. In every instance one should do everything medically and surgically possible to achieve healing from whatever disease condition he may have. Along with this, there should be concurrent prayer and the services of the enlightened Healing Church, such as the one in the quoted letter. When medical methods fail, the clergy must continue to uphold and uplift the patient. They can give him the constant support and optimistic viewpoint that—no matter what the situation—God has not failed;

that there is always the possibility of spontaneous remission or cure of the disease. This can always be the possible outcome for the patient who does not despair but continues to trust God.

Even when the physician decides to incorporate the truth of Christian healing into his practice, he is going to have apparent failures and disappointments. However, in those cases in which he does use this new philosophy of basic care, he will occasionally have cases in which results are spectacular and fascinating. This is not to say that the physician who adopts this philosophy will negate or diminish his scientific acumen. He adds to his scientific knowledge the necessary attributes of Christian belief and practice as recorded in the New Testament.

One such instance in my practice deserves mention. A middle-aged Jewish woman came to me for investigation of a mass in her right breast. She stated at the outset that the reason she had come to me was that I believed in prayer. Prior to the initial biopsy, the patient requested prayer. This gave the patient confidence and an inner sense of security prior to going to the operating room for what she realized might result in radical surgery. It also served to deepen the patient-doctor relationship. The mass proved to be cancer, and the breast was radically removed. Within a period of several months, and during the time when the patient was receiving X-ray therapy, she developed signs of spread of the cancer to her mediastinum and to her right lung. An X-ray report from the radiologist who was administering therapy stated that there was metastasis to the right lung with neoplastic abscess, which contained a fluid level within it. During this time, the patient became progressively more ill.

She was rehospitalized. Prior to the taking of additional X-ray studies, the patient again requested prayer. I recall going to her bedside one evening, taking her hand in mine, and praying for her. In the midst of the prayer, I asked Jesus to heal her. I realized at that instant that I had prayed in the name of Jesus, and I hesitated—feeling I had violated her religious belief—only to feel her hand squeeze mine as if to say, "That's all right, go ahead!" I finished my prayer, and much to my surprise the patient began immediately to improve. X-ray studies the following morning and additional studies the following week failed to disclose any residual neoplasm. The patient came to the immediate belief that Jesus is Messiah. What caused the healing is difficult to say, except certainly it must be stated that the factors of faith and prayer were of paramount importance. Love and concern for the patient and a refusal to become discouraged in the face of a most alarming situation must play its part. The body and the soul do respond to the spirit, and particularly when the human spirit is in harmony with the Spirit of God.

And he said unto her, Daughter, be of good comfort: thy faith hath made thee whole; . . . Luke 8:48.

7 - Cancer II

THE PHYSICIAN who would consider Jesus Christ's message of healing must re-evaluate his entire approach to patient care in the light of the Gospel message if he would develop a Christian orientation toward God and his fellow man. When he does this, hopeless conditions suddenly do not appear as devoid of hope as they did before. Optimism replaces pessimism. As a Christ-oriented physician views man's mortal enemy, cancer, this is also true. Cancer is the continuing dilemma of modern medicine and surgery. It is a disease with many faces and disguises, making it treacherous and insidious in its development. Eventually it becomes a multidisease entity which, as it progresses, involves physicians in many specialty groups. Physician and researcher alike today are looking for new therapies. The layman-patient is forced many times to his knees in prayer; so too, the doctor who so often sees impending death despite all his methods and surgeries. We live today in a world replete with many great advances which make the medical world of fifty years ago appear almost fictional, perhaps impossible. Surgical results in cancer are better today because of advances in medical treatment, surgical techniques, and medical technology; we better understand pathology and physiology. We have advanced in the fields of chemotherapy and radiation treatment of cancer.

However, many modes of therapy are not curative but are at best only palliative or life prolonging in their effect. It is wise, periodically, to view ourselves in the practice of medicine with a critical eye and hope that through wise criticism we may make progress and overcome complacency. Is there an assurance of hope in the individual cancer case which confronts us from day to day? In all honesty, it can be said that there is *hope!* There is also the chance that there may be no hope.

A patient who hears a physician's diagnosis of cancer has reached a tremendous and alarming crossroads in his life. The diagnosis of cancer may be categorized as a death sentence from which there is a possibility of reprieve. It is here that the physician and others caring for the patient must work together again to complete the care and to hold the patient up through the convalescent stages of his healing, or possibly through the terminal stages of the disease in the case of medical incurability. Even for the cured patient, the needed physical and psychological rehabilitation challenge the family, the doctor, and the clergyman. When the patient is medically incurable, the problem becomes much greater, and requires every resource of the physician's art, every ounce of love and understanding by the family, and prayerful support of the fellowship of the concerned in the Church.

Those interested in cancer patients must adopt a more personal interest in rehabilitation and the transformation of terminal-care facilities to centers of healing. Cancer societies should do more than simply supply information, dressings, beds, or utensils. Facilities for the instruction of the patient's family and the home care of the patient should be provided. Consideration also should be given to methods of alleviating the huge financial burden placed upon the families in some cases where the disease is painfully slow in its course. Closer cooperation between cancer societies, medical societies, and the Healing Christian Church is an important and critical necessity.

In view of the cases cited herein, it becomes apparent that along with all present areas of investigation, cancer should be investigated from the standpoint of the spiritual. The development of many neoplastic diseases bespeaks evil.

Cancer is something which the body itself produces. It is not analogous to infection, an invasion of the body by an organism attacking the body from without. The cancer cell is a cell of the body itself which one day, as a result of some influence, begins to become self-asserting. That cell then develops an inclination to live for itself at the expense of the rest of the body. It creates its own colony of similar cells. These cells are sometimes large and often dark in their nuclear and mitotic appearance. Cancerous areas are rapid in their growth and vital in their rapidity of multiplication. Once having established themselves in a colony, the cells may invade blood vessels, on occasion, or lymphatic channels, and not only spread by direct continuity but send out emissaries to other parts of the body to colonize and reproduce. These cellular masses increase in size until either the person who possesses such a disease is debilitated by the rapidity of the growth, or vital organs become involved to the point where they cannot function and death ensues.

The microscopic appearance of cancerous growth is one of destructiveness and a selfish disregard for needs of other cells which make up the harmony and function of the body. The cells seem to have no realization that, should they succeed in their purpose to take over, they will ultimately cause the destruction of the body which they inhabit to the point of destroying their own life in the process. This, if it can be termed a philosophy, is certainly the philosophy of the individual who decides to live for himself and, if necessary, to destroy those about him in order to achieve his own purposes. In other words, the basic philosophy of cancer is what might be termed that which has nothing to do with love, but has to do with personal or selfish gratification. The philosophy of cancer is satanic. If this is true, man must investigate neoplasms from the standpoint of the scientific and the surgical along with a multitude of other avenues. The basic spiritual aspect of the disease must be considered along with possible spiritual methods of its cure.

Not only does cancer have what seems to be a spiritual type of development, which is evil, but conceivably it also could well have, because of its malignant nature, evil etiological factors. Etiology means the knowledge of causes of illness. It may be that in the background of the individual developing cancer there is something—buried deep within the confines of the subconscious mind—of an emotional or spiritual nature such as hatred, fear, hostility, disappointment, heartbreak, or a number of other factors. These emotions are every bit as much spiritual as they are psychological. When unresolved, they can lie smoldering within the depths of the subconscious mind, cropping out subsequently with the development of cancer, mental illness, or other conditions sometimes called stress diseases.

At one time during surgical training, I was privileged to be a surgeon at a large prison. In the psychiatric unit of the prison was a young man who had become enamored of a girl whose family did not want to have him associated with their daughter. On one occasion, having left his work, he went to a bar to drink. After ingesting too much alcohol, he became angry and purchased a revolver. He then drove to his sweetheart's home and, drawing the gun, told the family that he was taking the girl with him. He took her in his car and drove off with her, only to be found sometime later and arrested on the charge of kidnapping.

He was tried and convicted. In prison he became extremely quiet and progressively more unresponsive. Whenever anyone tried to help him, he would become angry and uncontrollable. Eventually, he was placed in the psychiatric division of the prison which, at that time, had rather primitive methods of dealing with such problems. About this time he began complaining of a physical difficulty, and surgical consultation was obtained. This allowed me to see him. On examination, I found that he had a very large cancer of the lower bowel with involvement of the prostate and bladder, a situation which was entirely inoperable.

In this instance, we were confronted with the situation of cancer and the necessity of its surgical and medical management. However, there were serious psychological and spiritual factors which we never resolved because of our basic inability, in this instance, to see beyond the somatic problem. The physical problem became more and more acute as he was hospitalized over a period of months. Eventually he died. During this time, I was able to counsel with him on not only a psychological but a spiritual basis and was able to lead him to some measure of victory over his problem on the level of his spiritual being, as he became committed to Jesus Christ.

One wonders, in the development of his illness, had he sought spiritual counsel rather than going to a bar, and sought prayer and spiritual help in dealing with his sweetheart's family, if this entire process could not have been avoided. This is conjecture, but every physician who deals with cancer is confronted with similar problems which make him have concern that, perhaps on the level of the psychological and in particular the psychospiritual, we are missing a very important facet in the etiology and development of the disease of cancer, which should be more thoroughly investigated. Psychological studies have been carried out, but very little has been done in consideration of the spiritual. The error has been made in the past of considering the psychological and the spiritual to be the same. Not only should there be a consideration of the spiritual in the therapeutic and etiologic aspects of cancer, the entire problem should be subjected to deep spiritual consideration in all of its aspects.

Early in my surgical practice, I saw a young woman who had metastatic cancer of the breast. This young woman had the good fortune of being surrounded by a group of seriously concerned people in her church, who were praying for her. I was asked to see her not from the surgical point of view but in order to give her spiritual support. Her physician was in accord with this approach, since there was no other avenue of help for her.

The point of interest in her case is that spiritual therapy, in this instance consisting of prayer, both with her and by church prayer groups without her, did indeed help her in the betterment of her physical and emotional status. In considering the development of her illness it is interesting to note she had deep psychological problems, not only with her family prior to her marriage, but a basic rebellion against her family and against all spiritual considerations.

She had married in an attitude of rebellion. Her marriage

was an unhappy one in which she was never truly able to make a satisfactory adjustment. After development of her illness, during which the progress of the disease could not be stopped, her husband became concerned about her. When he started praying for her and loving her in a new and spiritually deeper way, she improved. Later however, her husband became interested in another woman; he stopped praying for her and being concerned for her, and the patient rapidly succumbed to her illness. The lack of love and replacement of love by resentment and indeed, hatred, are factors to be considered, not only etiologically but therapeutically, in cancer and any illness of man. Multiple studies have been carried out which demonstrate that animals and even plants surrounded by love and prayer will thrive, and those surrounded by hatred, resentment, argument, and similar factors, will wither.

In this day of scientific advances in which we are still striving so diligently to find the cause and treatment which will provide cure in the realm of cancer, it is well for the physician and the clergyman as well as the patient not to neglect the Gospel truth, that Jesus Christ is the Way and the Truth and the Life, and in Him lies hope, no matter how desperate one's situation may be.

It is unfortunate that cancer may be the factor which drives a person to his knees and to the necessity to seek the Lord in his life. This desperate aspect of the situation may not only save him unto eternal life, but there is the distinct possibility that such a conversion may result in healing. Herein lies the realm which, in my opinion, should be investigated on a deeper level, not only by the Church, but by those who are interested in the entire field of cancer and related diseases.

Jesus saith unto him, I am the way, the truth, and the life: no man cometh unto the Father, but by me. John 14:6.

. . . I am come that they might have life, and that they might have it more abundantly. John 10:10.

8 - The Infusion of Life

ONE OF THE most intriguing things about Christianity is its focus on life. A believer in Jesus Christ has not only the ground rules for abundant life on earth; he also sees how he may have eternal life. Eternal life is that life which the Christian individual lives now as he has come to Christ and accepted Him as Savior. Eternity is a measure of time, pertaining to the future from the present instant on. Through Christ we are now living in eternal life. "I write this to you who believe in . . . the name of the Son of God . . . so that you may know [with settled and absolute knowledge] that you [already] have life, yes, eternal life." (1 John 5:13) (AMP).

If we are already living in our eternal life, then we must see that it is simply the mind and flesh which are temporal. The spiritual man continues on in the eternal sense. The body and the mind (the psychosoma) are the perishable aspects of our Adamic nature. "And so it is written, The first man Adam was made a *living soul;* the last Adam was made a *quickening spirit.*" (1

Corinthians 15:45, italics mine). Any physician who has ever carried out an autopsy knows that the brain and the flesh are very dead after respiration and circulation cease. It is perfectly obvious that something has departed from the individual which is most assuredly spirit. That peculiar glowing, lifelike characteristic of the person is gone the instant death occurs. The ethereal spirit, the Christian believes, continues on to live forever with Christ. We know from the fact that Jesus was recognizable after His death and resurrection that we shall have, as Paul teaches, an incorruptible body, (". . . and the dead shall be raised incorruptible . . .") (1 Corinthians 15:52) that is to say a spiritual body which shall never see death or pain or disease, just as Jesus had.

This new creature (or creation) begins as soon as one has learned to begin dying to self and living unto Jesus Christ. This is the thrilling feature of Christianity. According to the Scripture, man does not enter into eternal nothingness nor does he live forever disembodied as an ethereal ghostly nebula. We shall, however, exist with our own bodies glorified and made more wondrously beautiful and functional.

It is most interesting to contemplate what Christ has made available to those who believe in Him. A person must stop thinking of his own possessions and of himself, and must take up his cross and follow the Lord Jesus Christ. He said man must be born again, "of the Spirit." If He is the Way, the Truth and the Life, we must truly believe this and begin to apply His way and His truth, as well as His life, in our life and practice.

For a doctor this becomes an important consideration, since doctors are in the life-conveying business. When a baby is born, it is imperative that the mother's life be preserved and the infant's, as well. At times many hectic moments go by before the first infant cry is heard or, on occasion, before the mother is resuscitated. These are times when all physicians know that life is a very tenuous possession, capable of being snuffed out or lost at any instant.

The life of Christ, lived to the best of one's ability by the individual, can infuse life into the life and surroundings of the believer. Wherever Jesus went, He conveyed life. Wherever the believer in Christ goes, he conveys life. There are people so devoid of vitality that they everywhere convey only sorrow and depression. Such cannot be the characteristic of the believer in Christ. His very life and being should emulate the life and being of Christ. Since the Savior and Healer of the world does indeed live and dwell within him, he must emulate Jesus as he lives out his personal imitation of Christ. He should be a conveyor of life in a very real way, just as Jesus was when He lived on earth, and just as He is as He dwells in the hearts of those who believe in Him.

There is an even deeper consideration, however, of the infusion of life than this. If the person who is interested in the Gospel of Jesus Christ reads the various narratives of the life of Christ with credulity, he must come to the conclusion that Jesus had a most striking ability when it came to dealing with those who were dead. One has no idea how many instances there were in which Jesus raised the dead, but there are instances recorded in the New Testament which must be considered. It does not appear that Jesus ever gave a person mouth-to-mouth breathing or artificial respiration of any sort, nor did He carry out cardiac massage. Rather, the same method was used by Him as was used by God at the instant of the creation of the universe. God spoke the universe into existence, "And God said, Let there be a firmament [the expanse of the sky] in the midst of the waters, and let it separate the waters [below] from the waters [above]." (Genesis 1:6) (AMP). Since God the Father spoke the universe and all of its contents into existence, it is not strange to see God incarnate, Jesus Christ, speaking life into the son of the widow of Nain, into Jairus' daughter, and into Lazarus.

The story of Lazarus is most important for the Christian to understand. I do not believe in diluting the truth of the narrative in John 11. It is with reference to the raising of Lazarus that Jesus stated John 11:25 & 26 (AMP), ". . . I am [Myself] the Resurrection and the Life. Whoever believes in (adheres to, trusts in, and relies on) Me, although he may die, yet he shall live; And whoever continues to live and believes in (has faith in, cleaves to, and relies on) Me shall never [actually] die at all. Do you believe this?" Immediately following this conversation, Jesus shouted with a loud voice, ". . . Lazarus, come forth." (John 11:43). The putrefying man who had been dead for four days came forth from his tomb wrapped in his burial garment!

As a physician, I prefer to accept the case history realistically, even though it does not seem possible that anyone who is decaying and putrefying could be brought back to life; however, if Jesus is God incarnate, He has the capacity of giving life even unto death. If this be true, physicians need to know more about Christ since they, and all medical personnel, are interested in the preservation and bestowing of *life*.

In the emergency rooms of hospitals and in first aid stations, on battle fronts, wherever emergency situations exist, the doctor and the nurse and those caring for the sick have the unusual sense, albeit at times rather a subconscious sense, of being involved in the area of the giving of life and even at times of the miraculous. There are those instances when one veritably despairs for the life of the person whom he is caring for, and in every physician's practice he has seen the moment of despair suddenly turn into the moment of hope. This may come as one plunges his hand into the chest cavity and begins to massage the heart and feels the flicker of life in his hand as the heart begins to assume its beat. There are those instances when the doctor, in order to reconvey life to an individual, may even break a bone or strike the chest of the patient, such an act creating such a reaction on the individual that life again resumes. I can remember an elderly Negro man who, at the moment anesthesia began, suddenly developed a cardiac arrest. This was immediately ascertained. Anesthesia was stopped and the patient was struck over the sternum forcibly with the fist. The heart immediately began beating, and the patient was sent to the recovery unit without surgery being performed.

These are instances where a definite act is done upon the body, causing a recalling to life of someone who, to all intents and purposes, is dead or is very close to being so. The patient who has severely hemorrhaged, as in a ruptured tubal pregnancy or a bleeding ulcer of esophageal varices, who comes into the emergency room bled out, unconscious and barely breathing, is an example where surgical treatment would almost appear miraculous. The physician, in such instances, will cut a major vein and start the infusion of blood or plasma. Every physician has, under such circumstances, seen his patient go from imminent death to life.

The infusion of life which was done through Jesus Christ, as in the case of Lazarus, was something of a higher dimension. What makes this so vitally interesting is the fact that Jesus stated,

". . . greater *works* than these shall he (the believer) do; because I go unto my Father." (John 14:12) (Parentheses mine).

For the physician who finds himself in that critical moment of despair when everything seems to be lost, it is indeed a joyous and wonderful thing to contemplate that, through Jesus Christ and through prayer in His name, despair may be turned into victory. Such a concept is hardly acceptable to the scientific mind, since there are no formulae or statistical bases upon which to establish such a consideration or hope. If a man is a spiritual being, and life, on the eternal scale, is a characteristic which is imparted to man through Jesus Christ, the physician—who is a conveyor of life and often the extension of the hands of Christ to the sick and suffering—must give more thorough consideration to the vital fact of what Jesus Christ can do for the physician himself.

There are a multitude of possible avenues of consideration, but two case histories come to mind in which the presence of the power of Jesus Christ spelled the difference between life and death. The author realizes that there is much room for discussion in both of the following cases, but insofar as is possible to determine, the factor spelling the difference between life and death, was the factor of belief in Jesus Christ, the presence of Jesus, the power of His Holy Spirit in one's life, and the imparting or infusing the life of Christ from one to another. Whatever a person is he manifests to others. If the individual is irascible and irritable, with a sullen, angry nature, this personality will have its effect and will spread to everyone surrounding him. By contrast, if he is joyful and happy and looks on the light side of things, that individual will create about him an atmosphere of lightheartedness and pleasantness. Similarly, when a person is living the power of Jesus Christ in his life, the power of Jesus Christ must manifest itself to those whom he contacts. On a greater scale, when one is confronted with emergency situations such as death, if Jesus Christ is *Life*, He can be imparted through the believing Christian into the life of a person, even conceivably, one who has died.

On one occasion, when our youngest son was two, I was astounded one morning to walk into the bedroom and find that he had apparently expired during his sleep. I had checked him just a few moments before, and found him feverish, apparently from a cold, but otherwise he seemed to be quite well; however, after the passage of a few minutes, on rechecking him, I found that he had no pulse and was not breathing. I can recall taking him into my arms and holding him up to God, and crying out, "Oh God, don't take my little boy from me!" I ran to the living room and, placing him across a footstool, I began to give him artificial respiration and to pray. After the passage of what seemed like an eternity in time, I felt him start to breathe and felt life come back into his little body beneath my hands. I took him immediately to the hospital; it was found that he had developed pneumonia, which condition cleared up without any residual difficulty within a few days.

In thinking about this wonderful healing and that God had privileged me to be a part of the healing of my son, I began to rationalize and felt that perhaps my son had just had an episode of apnea in which he had simply stopped breathing. It seemed that perhaps my personal concern and involvement with him could have been such that my clinical judgment was not as acute as it might otherwise have been. Perhaps I was unable to feel a pulse beat which actually was there. All these factors were coming into my mind as I attempted to reason it out. However, I could not deny the fact that, in response to my prayer, the Lord Jesus Christ had indeed given my little boy back to me, and this I could not, on the level of my spirit, deny.

Some weeks later, making hospital rounds, I heard an announcement over the loudspeaker system calling for any doctor to come to the pediatric department immediately. Since it was midafternoon and no other physicians were present in the hospital, I went up and was asked by the nurse in charge to declare a little girl deceased. Out in the corridor a mother stood weeping. In the room, a resuscitator worked feverishly to send oxygen into the lungs of a two-year-old girl. I noted that the child was receiving intravenous fluids and that a powerful blood-pressure stimulant was being given in the solution. I also noted that the oxygen tent in which the child had been placed was pushed aside and as far as could be determined, the child had died. There was no breathing discernible, and when I placed the stethoscope upon her chest, I could not hear a heartbeat. This had been the condition for some minutes. At this point, I asked the nurse to go and get a cardiac stimulant which I intended to inject. After the nurse left the room, and prior to my saying anything to the mother, as I listened to the child's chest, I placed by hand upon her head and was led to pray, asking God, who had given my little boy back to me, if he would give this little girl back to her mother. Such was my silent prayer. Before the nurse had returned to the room with the hypodermic, the child's heart had started to beat and she began to breathe. I went to the telephone and spoke to the pediatrician in charge of the case. His first question was whether or not I had secured permission for an autopsy. He told me the child had been seriously ill for several days with a terribly high temperature. Nothing that they had been able to do was able to resolve the condition. When he was told that the child was living, he gave the opinion that the child would not live, or if she did there would be something wrong with her mind. Nevertheless, the child did make an amazing recovery from that moment on.

There is something which we cannot define that God can give to those who believe in Him at times such as those recounted above. The light of Jesus Christ present within the inner man of the believer is such that it is transmissible to others even to the point of intervening in what otherwise might result in physical death. This same vital force transmitted into the life of the individual Christian is such that it can transform impossible situations into possible ones and darkness and hopelessness into light and optimism. This is a quality which life today needs desperately. The Gospel Truth needs to be taken from the churches and from the pages of the New Testament and lived out in the lives of believers, particularly those who profess and call themselves Christians. Were those who profess Christianity to begin to believe it, and to live it, certainly the world would know it within twenty-four hours. "Jesus said unto her, I am the resurrection, and the life: he that believeth in me, though he were dead, yet shall he live:" (John 11:25). If the power of Jesus' Resurrection is such, believers today should know what this power is. It should not be allowed to lie fallow in the institutional church; it should be applied in the lives of those who are Christians. This is particularly true for those who are in the practice of medicine or nursing or surrounded with difficult and oft-times impossible situations which in human terms are incurable or unimprovable. If Jesus Christ is God, and if His power is undiminished today, He who said that He would never leave us or forsake us, will be the factor in transforming the hopeless times of life into His divine and glorious hope.

These things I have spoken unto you, that in me ye might have peace. In the world ye shall have tribulation: but be of good cheer; I have overcome the world. John 16:33.

Fear not, little flock; for it is your Father's good pleasure to give you the kingdom. Luke 12:32.

9 - Fear and Pain

How SHOULD man consider pain? How should he pray about it, either in himself or in others? Can it be wrong to want deliverance from it? How did the martyrs bear the ghastly tortures they were subjected to? Is there a difference between cancerous pain and martyrdom, the latter being voluntary in most cases? Is pain an enemy or a friend?

Since these vital questions recur frequently in a doctor's life and practice, they must be answered not only from a medical standpoint, but also from the aspect of the individual Christian. I have just come from a patient suffering severe pain from an abdominal neoplasm. As I have known her over a period of several years, both in health and in illness, it is necessary that I analyze her reaction to her disease and its pain. This patient has endured previous suffering at the time of major surgery and has been able to buoy herself up through faith in God and through faith in her physicians. When she was in the hospital for surgery, she exhibited very little apprehension, tolerating hospitalization and aftercare without difficulty. Recently, however, she developed new symptoms. Another operation was performed which revealed an inoperable malignancy within the abdomen. This time the patient exhibited postoperatively much more apprehension about her situation, especially when she was told, at her request, that it was impossible to remove the growth and that she would require radiation treatment. As a Roman Catholic, she received the Sacrament of Extreme Unction. She was advised as to the efficacy of prayer and the need always of relying on the love of God, who sends health and does not send disease. When these things were done, she improved greatly. As disease continued and pain became more a problem, I observed in this patient's instance, as well as in others, that increasing apprehension and fear brought increasing pain. When I was with the patient, talking to her about faith and God's love and Christ's healing power, I saw the patient's apprehension decrease; as she became calm, her pain lessened. God's perfect love casts out fear, and as fear is cast out, pain also diminishes or becomes tolerable. In this particular connection, I have noted with Jewish patients and others who do not believe in Jesus Christ, that illness makes then conscious of the need for something greater than their own resources.

When one talks of the love of God and of the healing power of Christ, a wellspring of hope sends forth healing life into the weakening body. "Through the tender mercy of our God; whereby the dayspring from on high hath visited us, To give light to them that sit in darkness and in the shadow of death, to guide our feet into the way of peace." (Luke 1:78-79). Jarring pain makes the patient conscious of his body and of his own frailty. Man likes to project himself into a realm outside of his body many times, but pain acutely brings him back to reality and makes him aware of the framework in which the spirit and soul exist until death. The pain of medically hopeless illness so often brings the patient back to the reality of his body that he tends to live completely incarcerated by it, dwelling upon the physical abnormality in his body in every microscopic detail. This is not only often the case in patients with physical disease, but also in patients with neuroses.

When a hopeless situation is found, such as the patient I have described, it is necessary to instruct her on the importance of her body. She must know how concerned God is for our bodies, since He created them. Through the body, we are to reflect God's love, life, and beauty. It is necessary that, as the patient is constantly reminded of her body through pain, she accept its existence and the fact that she has something abnormal within the body which is causing pain. This is not to suggest that the patient become resigned to pain or resigned to illness, but the acceptance of the fact that the illness exists and that the body exists is important in its cure. Then, at this point, the patient can muster spiritual, psychological, and physical resources through prayer, the prayers of the concerned, and through the ministrations of the church. Healing can then occur even in hopeless situations. I have noted in my practice that the patient who is able to have spiritual therapy is enabled to rise above his illness and its pain, although still living in a sick body which he does not deny. When this is accomplished, the patient can get along with less medication, or even with none. Herein lies the concept of body object and body subject. Body object is the body with its illness as the primary and total consideration. Body subject is the body realized and accepted with its problems and illness, but as a part of a triune being—spirit, soul, and body—able to respond in health even in the midst of pain and disease.

Pain becomes worse the more one fights against it. One must never become resigned to pain, but must accept the fact that God has created nerves which feel pain in order to protect us from injury or to inform us that something is at fault. When disease causes irritation of these same protective nerve endings, one should not curse God for giving us nerves that feel pain, but should realize that the illness (which is not *of God*) is causing the problem. We then can take a step upward, knowing that God, who created our bodies, can give us strength and ability to overcome illness and pain. During childbirth, women find, as they accept the discomfort of labor contractions or *pains*, if they can cooperate with their pains, using them to help deliver the baby, they will minimize the discomfort and shorten the time of childbirth.

It is not wrong to want deliverance from pain. No one wishes to suffer, whether it be from a toothache, a gallbladder attack, a surgically inoperable cancer, or martyrdom. In all instances where pain is a component, prayer and closeness to Christ should be a primary consideration. If the pain serves to bring one closer to Christ, he can then find that, even through this discomfort, he is turning what superficially may be thought to be a curse into a blessing. Thus the sufferer ascends to a higher level of consciousness using the spiritualization of pain to be a stepping-stone toward God. The pain then does not become a stumbling block to the individual, but becomes a means of achieving greater spiritual heights. In the case of the toothache or the gallstone attack, the patient can seek and obtain surgical relief from the pain, although a certain amount of suffering may be required in the curing. The individual's prayer life and the prayer support of those who are helping, plus the spiritual ministrations of the church, will be of great help in bringing about rapid recovery. In the case of the inoperable cancer, the ideal treatment is prayer support, spiritual therapy, and loving medical and nursing care. This combination, added to personal prayer and belief, will serve to minimize pain.

With reference to martyrdom, usually only those who are unusually spiritual are subjected to martyrdom. It would not be martyrdom if one were not dying for faith and belief. It is, therefore, possible for the person who faces martyrdom to rely heavily upon the strength which the indwelling Christ gives him through prayer. He can thus overcome the tortures inflicted upon him through the overcoming of the world through Jesus. The pain of illness can similarly be tolerated by the sufferer's inner faith in the overcoming power and love of Jesus Christ.

When one prays for the patient who is suffering with pain, he should visualize the patient as being completely whole, surrounded by the love of God, indwelt by the love of Jesus, and empowered by the strength of the Holy Spirit. He should lift up those for whom he prays to the healing light of Jesus. This lifts the sufferer above pain and above illness; gives strength to the spiritual body and the love which casts out fear and takes away anxiety, factors which increase pain. The prayer for the presence of Christ in us and about us, and in the patient and about the patient, is the prayer of power and will make the problem of pain less a problem and more indeed a blessing.

Fear, whether of death or illness, is a tool of Satan used to defeat Christians and to bring about all manner of illnesses and emotional problems. Fear activates the disease process as well as symptoms. The Holy Bible states, "There is no fear in love; but perfect love casteth out fear: because fear hath torment . . ." (1 John 4:18). God is love, and therefore where God is there can be no fear, and where fear is there can be no God. Mathematically, this would be called an inverse proportion. The more fear we have, the less of God we have; the more of God we have, the less fear we have. Paul states in Romans 8:15, "For ye have not received the spirit of bondage again to fear; but ye have received the Spirit of adoption, whereby we cry, Abba, Father." Before one can receive the indwelling of the Holy Spirit, he must lay down his self, his intellectual being, as well as his ideas and traditions. Under these circumstances, one, full of the Holy Spirit, becomes convinced of the reality of Jesus Christ and His Resurrection Life. When this occurs, death is seen as something which has no sting, and the grave is seen as something which has no victory. Then the individual can state, as a French doctor friend of Tournier's did at the time of his impending death, when his physician wanted to give him medication to take away his pain, "Do not give me anything; I will not have anyone steal my death away from me."

We also need to recall the statement of Isaiah 4:5, "And the Lord will create upon every dwelling place of mount Zion, and upon her assemblies, a cloud and smoke by day, and the shining of a flaming fire by night: for upon all the glory *shall be* a defence." I sincerely believe that the glory of the Lord in the total being of the Christian is a defense not only against evil but also against disease and fear. If God protects the believer from illness, from poisons, from serpents (*see* Mark 16:17, 18), why then should he fear?

A physician might paraphrase Job 33:19-26 in the following way: Man is chastened with pain upon his bed, and all of his bones ache with heavy pain so that he may not desire food and is even revolted by it. His flesh shrinks away and his bones stick out. Such a man in his illness perceives his soul to be drawing near the grave and his life ebbing away. If there were a minister, a pastor, or one person in a thousand to show this man the way of uprightness and lead him to the Way, then God is gracious unto him and says, "Preserve him from death, for the ransom has been paid on Calvary's Cross." Then shall his flesh become fresher than a child's and he shall return in strength to the days of his youth. Then shall he pray unto God, and God will show him favor. He shall look upon his countenance with happiness, and his new righteousness within will he give forth unto his fellow man.

The same God through the same Jesus is the same today, as He was in the yesterday of Job, or the yesterday of the man with the withered arm, or the man who sat crippled, begging for bread at the gate called Beautiful. When should the Christian ever fear? Fear, death, sin, and illness were defeated at Calvary. Through belief in Jesus Christ, man is given peace and the ability to make his body subject, not the object, of his total being. When, through faith, he has learned this truth, one who believes can live above fear and pain even in the face of cancer or martyrdom.

And the Lord God caused a deep sleep to fall upon Adam, and he slept: and he took one of his ribs, and closed up the flesh instead thereof; Genesis 2:21.

10 - The Challenge of Unconsciousness

ON OCCASION there will enter into the practice of the physician or into the hospital, a patient who is unconscious or comatose. The immediate problem of unconsciousness, or coma, is of great interest to the physician. The patient in diabetic coma is a tremendous challenge to the internist. In the event that the patient has pathology in the central nervous system, the neurologist and the neurosurgeon diligently seek the cause of the problem and its proper treatment. As in all comparable situations, the acute problem is of much more interest to the physician than the chronic one. If it is impossible for the patient to be returned to consciousness, either through medical management or through surgery, he enters the category of chronicity in which both the medical staff and the nursing staff may give progressively less attention to his needs beyond the barest necessities. Such patients are often called *vegetables*. Nursing care is directed toward the physical needs of the patient so that bed sores do not develop, and normal respiratory exchange is maintained. Since there is no possibility of questioning the patient to determine his needs and desires, this type of patient becomes uninteresting and peripheral to the mainstream of both medical and nursing care.

Of similar challenge and interest is the patient who is unconscious as the result of anesthesia. Such a patient is like the patient who is unconscious for medical reasons whether it be an overdose of sleeping pills or a cerebrovascular accident. Under anesthesia, the narcotized cerebral cortex inhibits the patient's ability to cerebrate. With the body insensitive and unable to react except in a vegetative way, the surgeon can then proceed with the operation which is planned to correct a physical abnormality. With the patient unable to feel or respond, and with surgeon and the anesthesiologist concentrating on factors of the operation, it is amazingly possible to give attention so much to the procedure at hand that the patient as a whole is forgotten. Thus, during the operation, as the technical procedure goes ahead, it may be that the surgeon will discuss the entire realm of anatomy, pathology, and surgery of the condition upon which he is operating. He may quiz his interns or residents. On finding the abnormal process, he may describe it minutely, offering audible opinions to those in the operating room concerning prognosis of the condition. To a certain extent, all of this is understandable and reasonable.

There are situations which may not be as academic and enlightened as the instance cited. As the operation proceeds and things go well, there may be discussion of philosophy, sports, politics, or daily events without any regard for the fact that the patient is lying there asleep and conceivably, on the level of his spiritual being, able to absorb much of what is going on. If the surgeon is one who is vulgar or profane, it may be that the patient and observers are subjected to profanity or off-color stories. One of the great disappointments of surgery for me was to find that the operating room was not a sacred place; rather it was very much a workshop, at times devoid of true respect, particularly toward the individual who was anesthetized. It was amazing to me, as a young surgeon, to note the difference between the types of conversation carried on in the operating room when the patient was awake, as under spinal anesthesia, and when he was asleep under general anesthesia.

I once visited a large city where much surgery is done on the heart and major blood vessels. I elected to go to one of the hospitals to observe a heart operation. The patient was a little boy. During the early stages of the operation, the boy was already under anesthesia and as the cardiac bypass system was put in place, I noted with dismay that music piped into the operating room was anything but calm. I felt that music piped into an operating room should be most salutary for the patient and those who work in the operating room, particularly in such an operating room where there is great tension and much detail to be considered. However, this operating room was filled with frenetic, upsetting music. Coupled with conversation and the technical procedure, it created an atmosphere of bedlam rather than the peace and quiet which should be the atmosphere of an operating room. I noted that, when the surgeon got to the part of the operation in which the heart defect was to be repaired, he had the music turned off. Things at that time became quiet. Following the closure of the heart and the conclusion of the surgery, the operating room again became filled with conversation and noise. It was distracting to those observing the procedure and certainly must have been to everyone, especially the little patient, if only on the level of his subconscious or his spirit.

Another time I met a young woman victim of a cerebrovascular accident. She had been suddenly seized with a severe headache; within a few minutes she had lapsed into unconsciousness. She was sped to a local hospital where a neurosurgeon was summoned. In the operating room, openings had been drilled into her skull, a hemorrhage identified, and the hemorrhage pressure relieved. Following this procedure and a period of critical illness, the patient was left with a paralysis of half her body and an inability to say what she was thinking. Also, she reported that from the time she began to be aware after the stroke, she had a constant whirring sensation in her head.

At the time I met the patient, she had been ill more than two years. She attended a lecture I gave, in which I discussed my feeling that statements made in the presence of sleeping children, or of those anesthetized, were capable of creating problems subsequently in those who heard such conversations, albeit on the spiritual or subconscious level. She suddenly became aware that she remembered some of the things which had been said while she was unconscious during the surgery. For one thing, she remembered the sound of the drill as it penetrated her skull; she also remembered some of the conversation between surgeon and nurse. She recalled, for example, that the nurse had made a derogatory comment about her which, even in her state of unconsciousness, created an extreme feeling of resentment. When this fact came to the point of being recognized, she asked God to forgive her for her resentment and to wash away all of the effects of this resentment from her being. To her amazement, she immediately was released of anxiety and concern, and most amazing of all, the whirring sensation in her head suddenly disappeared, never to recur! She was also healed of her paralysis.

In the letter quoted from the patient with breast cancer, her surgeon had told her that the cancer had been completely eradicated by surgery. She said that she was extremely shattered some months later, when her surgeon told her that her situation was hopeless. She had previously been told that all the malignancy had been removed. She found, in conversation with friends, that the surgeon during the operation had stated that the situation was serious when he found not only the growth present in her breast, but spread into the lymph nodes of the axilla. Postoperatively, the patient experienced continuing apprehension and what she described as nightmares. No doubt the apprehension, the ill-defined fears, and the uncertainty which she experienced postoperatively were related to the imprinting of the negatives stated in the operating room upon the patient's subconscious mind and upon her spirit at the time of the surgery.

Once I was asked to see a child who had sustained a cardiac arrest approximately three months previously. This young girl had been unconscious and was living in a state of vegetation ever since the cardiac arrest and the time of being resuscitated. At the time of my examination, there was not a glimmer of consciousness. She lay thrashing about in her bed and looked very much like one trying to tear out of an envelope of darkness. She had a tracheotomy tube in her throat, a feeding tube in her stomach, and a catheter in the bladder. She was emaciated and severely, chronically, and terminally ill. Everything concerning her was despair. No hope was given to her or to her parents by the attending staff of the hospital. So far as could be determined the child had only a very short time in which to live.

In view of some of my convictions concerning the ability

to affect the spiritual being through conversation and prayer, it was my recommendation to the parents, to the nurses, and to attendants that nothing negative be further said in the presence of the patient. I felt there should be no prognostication over the patient, but that everything that was to be said should be optimistic. I encouraged the mother to visit the child frequently, to pray audibly with her, and to state such things as, "Karen, Jesus is healing you and you are going to become well." Besides the audible expressions of optimism, it was my feeling that the parents and those visiting the child should actually change their attitude toward her and begin to feel that she was not going to die, but that she was going to get well. In this context, they were encouraged that where Jesus Christ is, there is life and hope, and as they believed in Jesus, nothing would be impossible. They were also encouraged to say those things which were familiar to their daughter so that old patterns of thought and action could be brought to mind. With this change in attitude and approach, it was not very long before the child started to come out of her coma and began to recover.

When I visited Dr. Paul Tournier in Geneva, a member of the Bossey Medical Group was asked his opinion concerning prayer with the patient. After giving the matter some thought, he stated that he believed in prayer, but he also believed in helpful and health-giving attitudes on the part of nurse and physician. For example, he stated that in his practice many patients were given shock therapy for their mental conditions. He said, "Every bit as important as voiced prayer, if not more important, is what kind of eyes are going to greet the patient when he awakens from his shock therapy. Are they the eyes of love and care and concern or are they cold and impersonal?" Similarly, it might be asked, what kind of hands and arms care for and lift the patient from the treatment table to the stretcher and into his bed. What kind of an atmosphere of love and regard is there surrounding those people who care for the patient?

It is my considered opinion, after the observation of many anesthetized patients, that it is possible to implant negatives into the subconscious mind and conceivably into the spiritual being of the patient at the time of anesthesia or unconsciousness, which are of definite bearing on the patient's postoperative course and on the total outcome of whatever procedure has been used to correct his abnormality. Every bit as important as the technical aspects of the procedure are those factors which occur about the patient during the time of his unconsciousness. In this regard, it might be also stated that in one's home, one must never think that his children or any sleeping person is unable to receive and know spiritually what is going on during the time of sleep.

There are many situations, not only in the home, but especially in the hospital, where it is entirely possible for the patient to be adversely affected by those things which occur while he is not conscious. Therefore, consideration should be given to postanesthesia recovery rooms. Every effort should be made to make such areas as orderly and quiet as possible. Greater attention should be placed upon protecting the delicate sensibilities of the patient, particularly the patient who is unconscious. Conversations and noisiness in such a situation should be absolutely minimal. In this situation, as in the operating room, the use of quiet background music could conceivably be beneficial. Similarly, attention should be given to intensive-care units, which also are places in which the comatose patient may be placed. Again, in these areas, there is apt to be noise and confusion, plus the frenzy and scurrying about which are so common in places where life hangs in the balance. It is so easy in medicine and in nursing to be imbued with the problems at hand to the point where the patient's individual needs are pushed aside in order to take care of simply the major and critical consideration. In all such situations, as in the operating room, honor must be paid to the patient as an individual and as a human being. That honor must never be neglected, either as a result of expediency or neglect.

A friend of mine is a very deep-thinking psychiatrist. He has given considerable attention to spiritual factors in medicine, particularly in psychiatry. At one time he was discussing the fact that a patient who is asleep or unconscious is able to know what is happening about him. Ministers, he said in his lecture, should not be upset when parishioners fall asleep during sermons. Under such circumstances, he said, the message gets through to the mind unimpeded by extraneous factors such as sight, hearing, or wandering thought. This type of thinking has been utilized through what has been called *sleep therapy*. Certain positive thoughts are transcribed on tape recorders and played during the night beneath the pillow of the sleeping patient. Music has been similarly used to calm sleeping patients by using tape recorders to increase the calmness of sleep. It is interesting, also, to consider hypnosis and the fact that a susceptible subject will demonstrate he has received certain positive facts which he carried out in the post-hypnotic state.

It is entirely possible that certain positive or negative verbal suggestions which are given to the patient under anesthesia or sleep may similarly affect the person in terms of agitation or delay of postoperative recovery. Negative suggestions or statements, therefore, should be eliminated from operating rooms and from postanesthesia recovery rooms in the same way as they are not allowed in areas where a patient might hear them.

From the positive point of view, if the patient is told that everything went well during the operation and that he will make a wonderful recovery and will awake feeling well, it is possible that such suggestions could not help but ameliorate the patient's postoperative course.

I have found, in my own practice, where I am able to keep operating-room conversation down to a minimum and allow only positive statements to be made over the patient during the operation and following the operation, the patient does considerably better. I have found, in this regard, that when an operation is started with audible prayer, such an act creates a more salutary atmosphere in the operating room and positively stops peripheral conversation, particularly with reference to things which do not pertain to the operation itself.

By contrast, if an operation is not started with prayer and if the operating-room team is not oriented to God in some positive way, very often the operating room can become a place where there is much negative conversation and discussion of many topics irrelevant to the case. I should like to suggest that every doctor who professes himself a Christian follow the precept established by Ephraim McDowell, the first American surgeon to ever perform a laparotomy; Dr. McDowell began his first operative procedure with prayer. Similarly, Dr. Howard Kelly, of Johns Hopkins Medical School, always preceded his operative procedures with prayer. There is no more deeply spiritual discipline which the surgeon can utilize before operating. The prayer carried with it an absolutely positive suggestion for good and for benefit, not only to the patient but to members of the operating team. Following the operation, the patient should have the positive suggestion given to him that all has gone well, that God has answered prayer, that he has been protected through the operation, and that he is going to get well.

Investigations of twilight sleep have demonstrated that the patient can be interrogated under minimum degrees of anesthesia and suppressed thoughts and feelings of the subconscious can be ventilated. If such ventilation is possible at this point, it is conceivably true that positive suggestions can likewise be implanted into the patient who is emerging from and entering into anesthesia.

Certain specific instances are worthy of mention at this point. A prominent minister's wife went into the hospital for the delivery of a first infant. Shortly after arriving in the hospital, she began to hemorrhage and it was necessary for her to be taken immediately to the operating room where an emergency Caesarian section was carried out. During the procedure the patient was given blood transfusions in order to bring her out of shock. Not only was the patient in shock when she went into the operating room, but an anesthetic was administered. Following the operation, the patient was able to describe to the operating surgeon every detail of the procedure and much of the conversation in the operating room. Not only was there auditory memory, but she described the delivery of the infant, the fact that the surgeon had blood on the front of his operating gown, and many other factors. This latter fact is strange because a screen was placed between the patient and the operating team. So it was impossible for the patient to have seen the operation except by witnessing the procedure spiritually rather than psychologically. It can be theorized that the patient was under very light anesthesia, but insofar as could be determined by the patient's husband, and by the patient herself as she recalled the incident, she was in shock when she went into the operating room and was anesthetized with general anesthesia.

In the *Journal of the American Medical Association*, there was an interesting article from this standpoint. The authors described the case of a forty-year-old woman who was having a surgical operation for the correction of a cystocele and rectocele. The operation lasted two hours and fifty minutes and the anesthesia time was three hours and ten minutes. A general anesthetic was used along with the administration of neuromuscular blockade. The authors comment, "Despite this apparently uneventful anesthetic, the patient had a most unpleasant experience to relate to the surgeon and the anesthesiologist. She had been intermittently conscious and unconscious during the three hour anesthetic period. She volunteered the information that an airway had been inserted in her mouth and removed some later time. She reconstructed details pertaining to the discussion of the blood loss and the decision to start administration of the second unit of blood. She also experienced dull, unbearable, pelvic, lower back and perineal pain during much of the operation."

It is thus apparent that, even in cases albeit rare in occurrence, some patients are going to be aware of what is happening in the operating room. Even were the surgeon and the anesthesiologist to ignore the possibility of deleterious influence on the patient because of conversations in the operating room being picked up by the patient's spirit or subconscious mind, there is always the real possibility that such a case as the one described may occur and that the patient may indeed not only be hearing much of what is going on but may even be feeling what is being done.

An interesting comment is made by J. F. Artusio, writing in the *Journal of the American Medical Association*. "Quite by accident, one of my patients (under a light plane of anesthesia) responded to the spoken voice and indicated freedom from pain." Based upon this observation, Dr. Artusio taught a method of giving anesthetics in which the patient was carried along on very light anesthesia which he determined to be sufficient to knock out the pain sensation, but still of such a shallowness of anesthesia that he was able to converse with the patient and determine whether he was feeling pain or discomfort and, in general, was able to determine the patient's verbal and cerebral responses to the operative procedure.

These instances are cited primarily to serve as a basis of deeper consideration of the effects of unconsciousness, whether it be the operating room or a situation in which the patient is in coma. Anyone who is asleep or comatose must be treated as if he were awake and able to comprehend. Nothing negative should be said around him. If it is at all possible, spiritual factors should be considered such as prayer, and positive suggestions relative to the patient's recovery and his state, in general, should be given on the part of medical and nursing attendants. Under such circumstances, it cannot help but be of positive benefit to the patient and to everyone concerned, as the tenor of the operating room and the tenor of the sickroom respond to a higher orientation of doctor and nurse toward the human being whom they are treating and toward God who must truly be considered primary in all medical and nursing situations.

And one of the scribes came, and having heard them reasoning together, and perceiving that he had answered them well, asked him, Which is the first commandment of all? And Jesus answered him, The first of all the commandments is, Hear, O Israel; The Lord our God is one Lord: And thou shalt love the Lord thy God with all thy heart, and with all thy soul, and with all thy mind, and with all thy strength: this is the first commandment. Mark 12:28-30.

. . . Holy Father, keep through thine own name those whom thou hast given me, that they may be one, as we are. John 17:11.

11 - Synthesis

IN MEDICINE TODAY, as in theology, there is a tendency to divide man into a number of different categories. Those interested in theology concentrate upon man's spiritual being and those factors which relate to his spiritual being. This may be seen even in the sociological consideration, which is apt to be theoretical and ethereal. The minister who would leave his church to march in a parade, carrying a sign for some sociological objective, may do so more in an effort to identify with, rather than to actually be a part of, the group which he represents. He remains isolated from the real problem no matter how idealistic his desire may be. Similarly, in psychiatry, the psychiatrist lives and practices in a realm relatively isolated from medicine in general. Psychiatry as a field is also isolated by and large from theology. Insofar as medicine itself is concerned, instead of being one science concerning the body, it has been fragmented into various specialty fields. What is needed is a synthesis, or bringing together, of all the various concepts of man. Fragmentation destroys, whereas synthesis creates. It is necessary that man the human being be studied and treated from the standpoint of his whole being rather than in a piecemeal and incomplete manner.

Fragmented medicine is not in the best interest of the patient. Many examples can be cited. Recently I was asked to see a patient in the Southwest who was critically ill with cancer. When this man had first become ill, I was contacted by telephone. I had recommended a surgeon located near the patient. Shortly after the patient arrived in the hospital, the recommended surgeon told my patient that he was about to vacation in Europe, and since the patient had certain urological problems, he was going to call in a urologist. The urologist, an excellent man in his field, did not see the patient except from the standpoint of his specialty. Unfortunately, before the surgeon could return from Europe, the surgical condition, which had not been the matter of primary concern had created such severe problems that the patient had become critically ill. At this point, I was called upon. After examining the patient, I talked at length with his wife. She made the comment that, in discussing her husband's condition with the urologist, she had been told that the only aspect of her husband which he was qualified to answer questions about, or to take care of, was his urological system, and that she would have to talk to someone else regarding the surgical problem. Here-in lies the great problem of specialized medicine which grows greater as medicine becomes even more scientific. The patient becomes lost in the morass.

Fragmentation is altogether too common in medicine today. To counteract this problem, in some medical centers after a patient has been studied diagnostically, he is brought back to the original physician who takes all the consultation reports and laboratory studies and puts them together. Then he gives the patient and his family a complete picture of what is wrong. Too often, however in specialty-type situations, the patient is left confused and uncertain as to what is wrong with him. Beyond this fragmentation, there is a relative lack of consideration on the part of medicine in general to the psychological factor. Most physicians today think to only a minor extent about the psychiatric realm. They prescribe tranquilizers frequently and consider many of their patients to have nervous problems. Insofar as any true type of psychotherapy or attempt to get at the primary psychiatric problem is concerned (if this is the trigger mechanism of the patient's disease), this is rarely done. This attitude may be an outgrowth of the increased busyness of practice or it may simply be a desire not to be concerned about anything other than the immediate physical problem which presents itself. Certainly, caring for the immediate problem carries with it less necessity for the physician to identify with the patient or to become involved with him on any more than a superficial level.

Beyond the basic neglect of the psychological in medicine is neglect and disregard of the spiritual. In World War II, it was common for physicians to seek the chaplain's help in critical situations. This practice has become less and less apparent since the end of the war. Altogether too often the patient, as well as the physician, may not consider the spiritual except in those instances when death appears imminent. This is extremely unfortunate. A physician not oriented toward the spiritual who suggests a visit with the chaplain or perhaps even suggests that he himself pray with the patient may make the patient feel that his illness is more severe than he had thought—perhaps that he is about to expire.

A new and enlightened type of medical practice is needed in which the physician, even though a specialist, truly identifies on a deeper level with his patient and sees him as a whole individual, He must see that even something which involves the tip of the toe may, in its pain, its eventual consequences, involve the entire body. There is nothing that happens to any part of the envelope in which we live which can affect us only in an isolated area. We are aware that there are not only neurological factors which are involved whenever portions of the body are subjected to trauma or disease, but there are also hormonal and enzymatic considerations, lympathic and circulatory aspects, as well as psychological and spiritual factors which cannot be neglected or ignored.

The urgent need, then, is for synthesis! The physician must work in greater cooperation with the psychiatrist. Both the physician and the psychiatrist must see the clergyman in a new light as an ally and not someone simply to be called in for last rites, a prayer, or reassurance prior to death. Even as committees on religion and medicine are established in medical societies and in seminaries and psychiatric hospitals, the appointment of committees does not constitute a true answer to the dilemma of fragmented man. Unfortunately, there has not even been an adequate attempt to understand psychosomatic medicine. The psychiatrist is altogether too infrequently consulted concerning the patient with organic illness. He is rarely called to give strength and solace to the dying. Perhaps the reason for this is a basic feeling that the psychiatrist has become devoid of true consideration of the spiritual. The person who has centered his life in God and in Jesus Christ may fear that the psychiatrist may consider a vital orientation toward Christ equivalent to mental illness. A common concept in psychiatry is that troubled man turns to alcohol, sex, or religion for his solace. Religion is seen as a means of escape from reality. Religion is viewed warily and the spiritual aspect of man is rarely considered. Perhaps some of the reason for this is the fact that theologians have tended to go towards psychiatry rather than the psychiatrist going towards religion. Many ministers have established psychological counseling centers in relation with their churches, but these efforts have been primarily on the level of the psychological, often with the orientation toward Freudian psychiatry rather than any absolute or even tenuous relationship toward Jesus Christ. In the synthesis of man, there is a necessity for the minister or the theologian to reorient man toward Jesus Christ. In their ministration to the patient, they should not attempt to practice psychiatry or a form of religious psychiatry. They should practice logo-therapy—the treatment of the spirit of man—who can only be made whole through finding a meaning in life, such as provided by vital contact with Jesus Christ. To answer the anxieties and neuroses which plague intellectual man today, the psychiatrist must see that beyond the psychiatric is the spiritual; as he presents the psychiatric answer to the problem, he is only presenting a portion of the answer. The physician must see that he must not ignore the psychological and spiritual factors as he undertakes to create a well patient. To be well is to be whole!

In Switzerland, conversing with Dr. Paul Tournier and Professor Karlfried Graf Von Dürckheim, I once asked Dr. Tournier if successful healing after prayer were not something originating on the spiritual level and through the spiritual experience, as the mind, convinced healing had occurred, effected a body response in becoming well. Both Dr. Tournier and Dr. Von Dürckheim felt that the healing came through prayer; the spiritual being was healed through coming into harmony with God. The body was then healed as it responded to the spirit.

Then Von Dürckheim said, "The mind becomes healed as it, like a jealous little boy, lingers behind and waits to see what is happening, doubting and questioning whether healing can possibly have occurred." The mental area is the doubting, the questioning, and the worrying part of man. It is therefore, necessary for us to realize that there is a spiritual being, and that this spiritual being contacting God through Jesus Christ and the indwelling Holy Spirit, is able to overcome the mental nature of man, making the body whole. In the process, the mind is also made well.

It is interesting to read in the New Testament that Jesus always approached man as a primary spiritual consideration. Also, He did not heal man in the ordinary sense. To the woman with the bloody issue (*see* Mark 5:25-34), He did not say, "Your physical problem has been healed," but He did say, "Thy faith hath made thee *whole*" [italics mine]. In the story of the man who was born blind, the narrative does not deal with a man who has simply had his vision restored, but with a man who developed a deep spiritual belief in Jesus Christ, and who, despite the pressures of society and the negative attributes of those about him, decided to follow Jesus no matter what the consequences. It was more than just simply a return to sight; it was a manifestation of a total healing on all levels of his being. Many New Testament examples could be cited where the ministry of Jesus Christ was not simply that of the physician during a specific illness, but was presenting the kingdom of heaven to man. He gave encouragement to man: not only could he be healed of disease, but he could become *whole* in spirit, soul, and body, as he became a new person through Jesus Christ.

The synthesis required in the New Medicine is one which can come about through the avenue of a deep and real consideration of the part of a physician, ministers, psychiatrists, and man. They all must consider the place of the Lord Jesus Christ in life today. Jesus is the Synthesizer! He is the One who first showed how man can be brought together, rather than fragmented. It is wonderful to be able to treat physical illness with today's drugs and medications and operations. It is tragic, however, that so often we end up with a broken vessel. Psychiatry does not always put this broken vessel back together again. Psychiatry may teach a person how to live as a broken vessel, but Jesus, through awakening the spiritual and making a new creation of man, renews the psychological being and renews the physical being in the process! "And be not conformed to this world: but be ye *transformed* by the renewing of your mind. . ." (Romans 12:2, italics mine). This statement indicates that it is possible for an absolute renewal of the mental nature of man. This statement does not indicate the necessity for tranquilizers, or shock therapy, or psychotherapy, but does indicate that through Jesus Christ and coming apart from the world into the kingdom of heaven, which Jesus talked about, man can have a transformation of his mental being. Along with this there is the absolute fact that man, as he comes to Jesus Christ in the kingdom of heaven, can have a transformation of his physical being. This evolves as the spiritual being, the inward man, quickens to life through Jesus Christ.

The spiritual being exists as a small atrophic seed in man until it is nourished by the waters of the Holy Spirit. If the seed is fed by the forces of evil through immorality and the breaking of the Commandments of God, the inward man may develop as distorted, grotesque, and productive of sickness. On the other hand, if the spiritual seed is nourished by God through conversion, reading of the Bible and through concentration of the person upon those things which are good, he develops in the godly direction and becomes what the New Testament calls a new creature. Paul said it this way, "It is sown a natural (physical) body; it is raised a supernatural (a spiritual) body. [As surely as] there is a physical body, there is also a spiritual body" (1 Corinthians 15:44) (AMP). The spiritual body is not something which appears at the moment of death to go on to live with God forever if we have followed the precepts of God in our lives and not violated the Commandments. The spiritual body begins to live as soon as man realizes that his potential is that of being triune (logo-psychosomatic), through Jesus Christ, rather than biune (psychosomatic), without Him. John, in his first Epistle, said, "... it doth not yet appear what we shall be: but we know that, when he shall appear, we shall be like him. . ." (1 John 3:2). In this consideration, it can be seen that God, as He is portrayed in the Bible, is triune. That is to say that He has three natures: that of God the Father (the Creator and Organizer of the universe, "Elohim"); the Son (the manifestation of God in the form of man); and the Holy Spirit (the spiritual essence of God and of Jesus Christ existing potentially in man since Pentecost and existing in the world prior to Jesus Christ as an occasional gift to certain prophets and seers). Likewise, a man has the potential of being three in one. The spiritual aspect does not come into existence until he is born again: not physically, this time, but spiritually. The psychosomatic man, who has not been born of the spirit, is a partial and potentially a sick man, carrying within him the seeds of sickness and death. Triune man (the logo-psychosomatic man) would fulfill the category spoken of by John: "When He shall appear, we shall be *like* Him," three in one.

The New Testament writings of Paul are replete with this type of consideration. Paul, having had an absolute revelation of Jesus Christ in his life, was able to see this relationship of man in both its partial or psychosomatic considerations, and its whole or logo-psychosomatic ideal. Writing in Romans 12:1 (AMP), Paul says as he regards the body, "I appeal to you therefore, brethren, and beg of you in view of [all] the mercies of God, to make a decisive dedication of your bodies [presenting all your members and faculties] as a living sacrifice, holy (devoted, consecrated) and well pleasing to God, which is your reasonable...and spiritual worship." He states further (Romans 7:23-25) (AMP), ". . . I discern in my bodily members [in the sensitive appetites and wills of the flesh] a different law (rule of action) at war against the law of my mind (my reason) and making me a prisoner to the law of sin that dwells in my bodily organs . . . O unhappy and pitiable and wretched man that I am! Who will release and deliver me from [the shackles of] this body of death? O thank God! [He will!] through Jesus Christ . . . our Lord! So then indeed I, of myself with the mind and heart, serve the Law of God, but with the flesh the law of sin." In the following chapter, Paul gives the answer in that he speaks of the spiritual aspect of man and identifies the *mind of the flesh* as the mind of man without the Holy Spirit. The mind of man without the Holy Spirit is identified as the mind of the flesh which is death. In Romans 12, Paul beseeches that men be transformed (*not* transform himself) by the renewing of the mind. "Let this. . .mind be in you which was in Christ Jesus" (Philippians 2:5) (AMP). Psychosomatic man is described in Romans 7 and the fulfillment of man showing how man can be whole through the indwelling of the Holy Spirit and the coming-alive and growth within man of his spiritual being is described by Paul in Romans 8.

When man is ill, he can recover through fragmentational medicine which typifies today's average medical practice. Such medical practice breaks down when the illness is beyond its knowledge; for example, in terminal cancer, multiple myeloma, advancing multiple sclerosis, and many other similar conditions. The new medicine which was first spoken of by Tournier and alluded to by Dr. Viktor Frankl, logo-psychosomatic medicine, does not break down under such circumstances but becomes even more potent and real. The doctor who wishes to attend the whole patient certainly does not summon another physician, or even a minister or a prayer group, to pray for his patient until he himself has ministered to his patient's spirit. That there is truly a ministry in the practice of medicine is even spoken of in the "Principles of Medical Ethics of the American Medical Association," 1949 Edition, page 4: "The profession of medicine, having for its end the common good of mankind, knows nothing of national enmities, of political strife, or sectarian dissensions. Disease and pain the sole conditions of its *ministry*, it is disquieted by no misgivings concerning the justice and honesty of its clients' cause, but dispenses its peculiar benefits, without stint or scruple, to men of every country, and party and rank, and religion, and to men of no religion at all." It is thus seen, in the principles of medical ethics, that medicine is truly a ministry, and that as its ministry is given out to people of all sorts, it is the common good of mankind which is being sought. There are no conditions to this ministry except the fundamental needs of the sick patient.

Regarding expansion of the ministry to the whole patient, there are some areas of difficulty for which it is necessary to call in spiritual help from chaplain, minister, or prayer group. Possibly, well-meaning attempts of people lacking medical orientation may actually do harm; alarm or concern can be injected as a result of honest attempts to be helpful. Such dangers could be avoided if those wishing to pray, whether layman or minister, would contact the patient's physician for advice and suggestions. As medicine is practiced today, there would be certain misunderstandings, but as medicine grows in the direction of the spiritual, the physician will find that he can be of great assistance to the minister if he will take a small amount of his time to orient him toward the patient's needs. Certainly, the physician is the one who is oriented toward the needs of the whole patient, and if anyone is going to pray, it truly should be he, if he indeed has the spiritual orientation and the conviction that ". . .with God nothing shall be impossible." (Luke 1:37).

This is a sort of discipline different from writing out a prescription, applying a bandage, carrying out a surgical operation, or administering shock therapy. There is a deep personal involvement of the physician with his patient on the level of the spiritual with consequent effects upon the mind and body. This is present whether the physician or surgeon chooses to recognize it or not. The conscious involvement of the physician on the level of the spiritual carries with it a far deeper implication than the calling in of a clergyman to pray or to administer sacraments. When the physician gives credence to the power of God and the power of prayer, there is a tremendous bolstering of the faith of the patient. Such an act or statement of belief on the part of the doctor does much to bolster the patient's faith and can carry him through any trial no matter how serious the course that lies ahead.

As the team of physician, psychiatrist, and clergyman ministers to the whole man, the place of the clergyman and others must be considered. *Others* would include those laymen having a true ministry of intercession and prayer for the sick. Those who would desire to minister to the sick should be oriented to the basic psychological needs of the patient; they should be sensitive to the status of the patient, both physically and psychologically. In recent years there have been institutes of pastoral care established in major medical centers where hospital chaplains teach clergymen and certain laymen the art of ministering to sick patients. This is a great step in the right direction, but still there are many who come uninstructed to minister spiritually to the patient. Strangely enough the ministry of the uninstructed very often carries the potential of more good for the patient than the ministry of those who have had much instruction. The reason for this may be that instruction carries with it the potential of diluting the faith of the minister to the point where he develops a greater belief in medical science than he does in his spiritual ministration. This has been my personal observation. The minister needs to see that he has truly a field of his own in which his duty is simply to present Jesus Christ and the power of His Holy Spirit to the sick patient. It is not his place to fill in for the psychiatrist nor to give medical advice. He is not to prognosticate nor to carry sorrow or worry to the patient. He must carry joy, confidence, and hope, which are the normal attributes of the ministry of Jesus Christ. The various ministrations carried out towards the patient will vary according to religious practice. As a physician, it is my conviction that the method of ministry is of little concern so long as the minister or the person who is praying remembers that it is not the ministration or the method which heals or gives solace, but it is the presence of Jesus Christ in the act of prayer or in the visit which is of primary importance.

In many churches there are what are called healing services in which various methods of ministering to the patient are practiced. The physician should be aware of these services and their potential benefit for his patient. If medicine in general were more cognizant of such ministries and areas of help for the patient, they would be utilized more frequently. The healing services of the Church, whether they be prayer, anointing with oil, the laying on of hands, or spiritual counsel, are all scriptural methods which are legitimate and proper. Again, they should be utilized by those ministers who have deep discernment of the physical and psychological as well as the spiritual needs of those who come to them. The area of cooperation which is needed in medicine today is not just one of hospital ministry but likewise when the patient is out of the hospital. The enlightened physician may find that his own personal attendance in the church at the time of healing services may be of great strength and benefit to his patients who attend such services.

Reverence is a needed virtue in life today, especially in medicine and nursing. Surgeons are familiar with this virtue in what is termed *reverence for tissue*. Reverence for tissue is that type of surgical technique which handles the tissues of the body at the time of surgery with great delicacy, avoiding injury and trauma at the time of an operation. A surgeon with reverence for tissue has patients who do well following surgery and who do not have the stormy, difficult, postoperative courses of patients treated by surgeons who are rough and indelicate in their handling of the body tissues. How can there be reverence for tissue if there is not reverence for the human being, and how can there be reverence for the human being, if there is not reverence for God? Many surgeons who have not given deep consideration to these matters have an orientation toward the person of the patient and towards God manifest through their actions, if not through their verbal expression. When a surgeon sees that through his natural love for his art and his patient he is close to God, he can embrace Him whom he has known as close Friend, with whom he has always worked, not knowing who He was.

It is a common belief on the part of physicians that a consideration of the human being is of absolute importance. On one occasion, when I was a medical student, I was with a group of senior students making rounds with the renowned surgeon, Dr. Frederick Coller. The patient being examined and discussed was on a large, open ward with a screen pulled about her. Approximately twenty medical students and members of the house staff were present. Something was said by one of the residents to Dr. Coller regarding the patient and, with this, the patient began to weep with evidence of great mental anguish. The young physician who was taking care of the patient stood at the patient's side, unable to do anything to give her solace. Dr. Coller looked deeply at his resident surgeon and stated, "It is your duty as a physician to always comfort the patient, so it is your responsibility now to comfort her."

Certainly, with the many successful surgical and technical procedures that we are able to perform on the patient today, there remains always the necessity to give comfort and succor in the times of mental and spiritual torment, which invariably go along with any illness, no matter how minor. An illness is always a threat to the person. The only solace to an ill person may be that given by the physician who stands in the position of the comforter. For those physicians, surgeons, and nurses who will read the New Testament from the point of view of the Medicine of the Whole Person, it will be seen that the precepts of the New Testament Christianity are admirably applicable to an enlightened medical, surgical, psychiatric and nursing practice. It gives comfort and solace to the patient in a way not possible through absolute preoccupation with technological considerations, which will always be cold and sterile until the person and the spirit are considered. As God through Jesus Christ enters the heart of doctor and nurse, and as medicine, psychiatry, and the holy ministry unite in caring for the sick and hopeless, the fragmentation of man will cease; not only will man become whole, but those who minister to the sick will also! ". . . that they may be one, as we are" (*see* John 17:11).

Synthesis II—A New Medicine

"And he that sat upon the throne said, Behold, I make all things new . . . " (Revelation 21:5).

Medical practice like life, is an ever-changing panorama. Recent medical terminology has grasped General Jan Smuts' word *holism*, and from it has been launched a new realm of medical thought and practice. Whether or not Smuts' concept of holism is at all part of what is termed holistic medicine appears to be of little consequence. The field of holism in medicine now must be considered and applied to already overcomplex and scientifically top-heavy medical practice. In addition, the patient also must have some understanding of holism, since it will doubtless become more and more an alternative method of medical care for him and for his family.

There would appear to be little help in introducing other alternative terms in this consideration. The whole-person concept in our early writings has been refashioned *holistic medicine, wholism or holism.* The most biblical and definitive term regarding the whole man and his life is *logo-psychosomatic medicine.* Both Viktor Frankl and Jan Smuts would be comfortable with the logos as an expansion of psychosomatic medicine. In this writing, I deal with holism as a logo-psychosomatic consideration of the whole person—spirit, soul, and body. This I feel is a logical extension of Smuts' original writings and is the reasonable expression of Smuts' ideas as modified through the writings of great Christian scientists such as Tournier and Carrel. Of holism, Jan Smuts writes, in *Holism and Evolution,* "And Holism, standing on that high level of attainment in the human, points the way to the future, and shows that in wholeness, in the creation of ever more perfect wholes, lies the inner meaning and trend of the universe. It is as if the Great Creative Spirit hath said: 'Behold, I make all things whole.'"

As the world and the universe become better understood, man and his ideas continue to evolve. So does the care of the sick patient and the philosophy of health in general as the Creator Spirit reveals His great plan. Thus medicine is looking beyond the psychosomatic, to the creation of a new medicine, utilizing all of the best aspects of previous practice and incorporating revitalized and renewed thought concerning man as not only mind and body (temporal being) but also spirit (eternal being).

It may seem strange that America, with its apparent fascination with medications and medical gadgetry, is becoming disenchanted with medicine in general.

First of all, there is the continuing pressure from organized labor and the politically liberal segment toward the socialization of the governmentalization of medicine. This is nothing new, but has been a matter of evolvement over the past forty years, encompassing Medicare, Medicaid, and other government programs. The next step in the process could be some form of national health insurance. The cry for change in medical care has come about because of the failure of medicine, as ordinarily practiced, to meet the care needs of the majority of the people, particularly in a way which they can afford. Also, there is a growing resentment on the part of Americans in general against the high cost of doctor and hospital care, coupled with a sense of lack of compassion and personal interest of physicians and all who contact the sick.

On the grass-roots level of patient care, people have already begun in various ways to effect changes for themselves and their families. As an example, the patient inquiring of his doctor regarding vitamins, hypoglycemia, the use of alcohol socially, and abortion, could well find that the physician does not really believe in the use of vitamins, he doubts the entity of spontaneous hypoglycemia, he uses and often prescribes the use of alcohol, and believes in and advises abortion on demand. As a result, most Americans prescribe their own vitamin intake through health-food stores. They also modify their own diets for their self-diagnosed hypoglycemia (whether they have it or not). They join Alcoholics Anonymous or stop drinking on their own. They also join right-to-life groups, and view most physicians as enemies to their cause.

Feeling that life expectancy has not increased, despite immense hospitals and immense cost and a plethora of doctors and all kinds of ancillary personnel, the potential patient looks for other avenues. He looks for ways and means of increasing the quality of his life from day to day. He is also afraid that he might eventually find himself in that place called a hospital, where he may have little or no say about what is done to him and where it could be that almost no one would care.

As a result, the patient himself is requesting a new vital consideration of preventive medicine. Because legitimate physicians are loathe to change in new directions, the entire area of wholistic (holistic) medicine has attracted physicians peripheral to the main stream of medicine. In the entourage of those in this area of endeavor are those who have written such articles as "Occult Medicine Can Save Your Life" and a physician described as "The most widely used of the clairvoyant diagnosticians in the country." Utilizing biofeedback techniques and mind-control methodologies, the entire area of holistic medicine is springing up as an alternative method of health care and health maintenance.

In addition, much of the impetus for the hospice movement in America has come from clergy, nurses, and patients. In November 1976, when Elizabeth Kubler-Ross and Dr. Cecily Saunders (among many nurses, physicians and clergy) met in Montreal to discuss hospice, there was basically only one effective hospice in America. This was the New Haven Hospice, under Dr. Sylvia Lack. Most other endeavors at that time were purely embryonic. Since that time there has been a virtual explosion of interest in the creation of hospices across America for the care of the terminally ill. Key to the hospice philosophy is the belief that there comes a time when the kind of care and treatment afforded terminal patients in ordinary hospitals must cease. The emphasis in hospice is upon high-personal, low-technical patient care. Somehow the hospice movement also represents a rebellion against the kind of care ordinarily given to the patient in our depersonalized medical institutions.

Additionally, lay groups are springing up across America. There are those who advocate alternative methods of cancer treatment. There are acupuncture clinics. The patient may elect to go to a hypnotist. He could also elect to have psychic surgery or psychic healing. He could decide to try Therapeutic Touch or chiropractic treatment. The area of occult or spiritistic medicine is unending in its variety and complexity. Investigations are being carried out by those interested in the methods of witch doctors and those involved in voodoo and other satanic rites.

For the person who is not involved in the care of the sick, and particularly of the hopeless patient, this is amazing and shocking. However, it is true that the patient or his family will go to almost any conceivable length in order to obtain relief or cure for himself or his loved one. If modern American medicine were succeeding, we would see no such problem on the contemporary scene. We see, however, a proliferation of every kind of treatment method, a startling indication that somehow we have not been succeeding. Some may say that we have failed.

This may seem an extremely harsh assessment of medical care practices, but the physician finds that he can never correctly treat a disease until the correct diagnosis is made. Having been in medicine as student and doctor for over fifty years, I have had an opportunity to view medical practice, to analyze it, and beyond that, to pray about it as a Christian filled with God's Holy Spirit. My conclusion has been that medicine and nursing in America (and this includes the entire Western world) has failed in only one major respect: We have ignored Jesus Christ, His holy Word, and His holiness in our professions. All that is necessary to correct the major problems now faced by medicine and the patients it treats, is to make medicine spiritual.

We must have a believing Church, empowered by the Holy Spirit, practicing the spiritual gifts of healing. People must hear the truth that "Jesus heals today." This should be the witness of Christian physicians, who should tell their patients that "we may appear to be healers, but it is God who makes the sick whole." Medicine and nursing must be seen as holy ministries, utilizing believing prayer as their greatest therapeutic instrument of compassion. If the Church were seen as a center of health maintenance and healing, and medicine as an adjunct to the Church, modern medical practice would begin to see changes in patient attitudes, mortality, and morbidity statistics. For this to happen, there needs to be not only a spiritual revolution in medicine, nursing, and psychiatry, but also in the Church.

Where there is no vision, the people perish: . . . Proverbs 29:18.

12 - The Experiment

IN THE LABORATORIES of hospitals and institutions across the world, many varying experiments are being conducted in an attempt to study man and various aspects of man's disease and its treatment. More research is being conducted now than at any former time. As the results of this massive research are made known and as they are applied to patients, man should become healthier. As these advances are made daily, they are often applied in situations which are inadequate, oftentimes disturbing and not always health-producing. With all medical and laboratory factors controlled and superior in quality, the patient can find himself displeased, anxious, and unable to become well because of the hospital environment. An experiment in hospital patient care which applies the principles of the Medicine of the Whole Person has been needed.

It became apparent in the 1950's to some of us that there should be a hospital in which a new type of basic orientation of the facility itself should be attempted. Such a hospital would be oriented to a deeper concept and discipline of medicine through a total belief in caring not only for patients physically and psychologically but also spiritually. Such a hospital, it was theorized, should be centered in the Person of Jesus Christ and the power of His Holy Spirit.

Concerning hospital staff, the personnel in all departments should be oriented toward Christian principles, and this should be true, not only in all of the nursing divisions, but also in the orderlies, nurses' aides, diet kitchen, and ancillary service, including laboratory, X-ray, and physical medicine. It was also seen that the personnel in administration in the business office as well as the medical staff required a similar orientation toward a deeper consideration of the patient than is ordinarily understood. This orientation should be *lived* on the part of the personnel of the hospital in every activity, placing the patient in the position of primary consideration.

Such a hospital would possess an atmosphere of care and concern which should be the atmosphere in which healing could best be achieved. An attempt should be made to keep out such noisiness as television and radio. Noisy patients should be isolated where they do not disturb others. Loud talking and anything disturbing should not be allowed. The use of music would be vital. Music should be carefully screened to insure a salutary and comforting rather than upsetting effect.

Chapel services should be held in the hospital and be open to all patients with no attempt to point the patient in the direction of any one religious denomination. In the chapel services the truth in the New Testament concerning Jesus Christ and the power of the Holy Spirit should be considered primary. In conjunction with the chapel, a library should be a vital part of the hospital. There such decor as a fireplace and comfortable lounging area should be provided so patients can be quiet and comfortable in a homelike atmosphere. Meticulous cleanliness must be absolutely essential. Even though the patients many times are elderly and victims of strokes and neurological disease, the odors of such illnesses should be eliminated through absolute cleanliness and through the use of air-filtration mechanism.

Hospital personnel of such a hospital should receive instruction that they should present Jesus Christ to the patient—not through verbal expression, necessarily, but more through what their eyes and their hands and their attitudes speak. The Bible should be present on every bedside stand for every patient to read, but Christianity should not be forced upon the patient. As the patient begins to wonder why the hospital is different and why there is so much love and care and general improvement in his condition, he will naturally be led to ask what the difference is.

Vital physical medicine is also a necessity wherein not only the usual types of therapy would by utilized, but such therapy would be given with prayer and with a concern for the spiritual being of each patient. Patients' rooms should be accessible to the out-of-doors, to fresh air and sunshine, and gardens, and every room requires decoration with soothing colors and those which bring comfort and happiness to the patient.

Such a hospital did indeed come into existence as Christian Medical Foundation, Incorporated, administered a new convalescent and rehabilitation facility in Medford, Oregon, in 1964. For two years, Christian Medical Foundation, through staffing and through bringing about the conditions described above, was able to perform an unusual ministry to patients, many of whom were considered medically and surgically hopeless. This experiment was not carried out in a laboratory or in a large university center. It was an experiment in the Medicine of the Whole Person, carried out because many consecrated and dedicated people wanted to see if it would be possible in our time to create a hospital for the whole person. In the two years of this experiment, it was proved that such a hospital is feasible and can produce astounding improvement in patients who, to all intents and purposes, are hopelessly, chronically, and terminally ill.

Various examples of this could be cited, but certain cases were outstanding. Although it is difficult to make a statistical measurement of such factors, the clinical improvement of patients in the categories represented is significant. One patient dying of cancer of the breast was almost comatose at the time of admission to the hospital; she remarked to her husband shortly after entering the hospital room, "Oh, I like it here." She then lapsed back into deep coma. The nurses and hospital personnel who cared for the patient talked to her even though she was unconscious and encouraged her not only insofar as her physical being was concerned, but also her spiritual being. She was surrounded and uplifted on the arms of absolute care and total concern. She was the center of prayer on the part of the entire hospital as morning prayers were said and as the personnel performed their duties of the day. Within a short time, the patient came out of coma and gradually, despite the generalized spread of cancer through her body, became well enough and strong enough to insist upon going home. This patient was brought to the hospital to die, but something happened as a result of the care and loving concern manifested toward her so that she did not die, but developed great peace and a lack of pain, which had been severe prior to her admission to the hospital. Even though the patient ultimately died, she never had a recurrence of pain, and it was never necessary for her to reenter the hospital.

Another terminal cancer patient who was admitted for care became progressively more and more interested in what it was that she felt in the atmosphere of the hospital. On one occasion she said, "If I could only reach out and touch what I sense is present here, I know that I would be healed."

A patient who had cancer was admitted to the hospital for terminal care. She was extremely depressed and without hope. As she entered her room she requested that the curtains and drapes be drawn to keep the room dark. She spent most of her time in bed and was very quiet, tending to spend much of her time in sleep. As the staff ministered to her, not in words but in acts and in being, and as the atmosphere of the hospital surrounded her with love and care and peace, the patient began to open her drapes and take notice of the flowers and the garden and the beauty of the surrounding countryside. Day by day, instead of getting worse, she became better. On one occasion a member of the family came to the hospital administrator and in great concern said that he did not know what we were doing to his mother-in-law, but he wanted it stopped because he and all of the members of the family had been informed and were aware that the patient was going to die and they expected this. The patient expected this and they did not want her to come out of the hospital only to get sick again and die later. When it was explained to the man that nothing was being done except to surround the patient with loving care, he became pacified. Gradually, as the family became aware that the patient's general health and attitude were those of wholeness rather than illness, their despair and anxiety turned to joy. At this time, the patient requested to be discharged from the hospital and was sent home. Her eventual outcome is unknown at this writing but suffice it to say that in this instance, as in other instances, those patients who came to the hospital in despair and terminal, found life and hope as the healing love of Christ was presented to them. No cancer chemotherapy or other modes of specific medical treatment were utilized in the hospital since patients receiving such therapy were transferred to other facilities. The only modalities of therapy administered to patients in the hospital were excellent nursing care, adequate diet, and the ordinary medications for pain relief and tranquilization as ordered by the personal physician of each patient.

At the time Christian Medical Foundation began its experiment at the hospital, there was a young man who had been in various hospitals for approximately five years. This young man, in his early twenties, had been in a truck struck by a train. He suffered severe brain damage and multiple extreme injuries. When first seen, he was bedridden and emaciated. There was very little ability to communicate on any level and he was basically in a state of increasing vegetation.

As a result of the constant care and concern on the part of the dedicated nursing staff, the patient gradually was able to be taken out of bed. Through the efforts of the nurses, it was not long before he was able to stand and be fitted with a brace and then to begin to ambulate. His entire being at the time of our first contact with him bespoke of catabolism, the tearing down or breaking down of the body structure. Through love, total care, and proper diet, soon the emaciation had disappeared and his body configuration and general attitude bespoke anabolism, or the building up of his body structure.

Certainly, one of the great anabolic factors in healing is love and hope and the knowledge that somebody cares. To be left in a bed with the prospect of death with no hope is a tremendous catabolic, or destructive, influence upon the body and mind.

One day an elderly woman was admitted who was extremely irrational and unmanageable. Because of her noisiness and confusion, she had to be placed in a quiet room where she would disturb no one. It was necessary to secure the door to her room at all times. In an attempt to get out, she would spend long periods of time pounding at the window with her slipper. She successfully managed to remove the sliding doors of her closet and everything that was not absolutely secured in the room was soon torn apart.

This patient was the grandmother of a minister's wife who had brought her to the hospital, feeling that the ministry of Christian healing could help her. During the patient's early hospital stay, she was the subject of constant prayers on the part of the hospital staff. Nothing was done in this regard to the patient in a direct manner; she was simply held up in prayer constantly by everyone of the hospital personnel. Gradually it became apparent that she was becoming more tranquil; soon she stopped all noisiness, became quiet, and spent most of her time quietly singing to herself and praying. No shock therapy or drug therapy was necessary. In fact, the drugs which were prescribed at the beginning of her hospital course were gradually discontinued, and as they were discontinued, the patient became more peaceful. In her instance, it was demonstrated that prayer and loving concern on the part of the hospital staff can calm even a disturbed, senile patient.

There were many instances of patients who came into the hospital for terminal care, distraught and full of fear at the time of their entry. One elderly man with cancer of the lung entered in this frame of mind. Gradually, as he was surrounded by the atmosphere of the hospital, he became peaceful and quiet. He asked for help from one of the nurses. The nurse told him what it was that was different about the hospital, and he made the comment that if this was what Christianity was, he wanted to know more about Jesus Christ. He soon became a Christian and became born of the Spirit. As this occurred, his need for medication became minimal and even though physical healing of his illness did not occur, he became a whole person and died in peace without fear.

Many of the patients in such a hospital are those who are elderly and at times senile. It was noted that, as these patients were placed in an atmosphere of peace, where they were surrounded by beauty, their agitation and disturbance became less and less apparent. In many instances, these patients became wonderfully adjusted and presented none of the problems which had been present before entering the hospital. They were able to participate in occupational therapy activities and were vitally interested in the meetings in the chapel and in the discussion groups. These patients, who are of increasing concern in American medicine today, cannot be helped in the ordinary nursing-home situation. However, in such an atmosphere as was present at the Christian Medical Foundation Hospital in Medford, there was in all instances an absolute improvement in patients cared for by the staff with this new and vital concept of medical and nursing care.

Although it is impossible to give a statistical analysis of all the cases which were cared for during the period of the experiment, it is my conclusion that Medicine of the Whole Person, in such a hospital situation, albeit one where at times the most difficult type of patients were being cared for, is a type of medical and nursing practice which is extremely salutary and productive of healing. This is an absolute departure from what is seen in the average hospital today where, as the scientific aspect of medicine becomes more and more pronounced, the patient becomes just a small part of a great machine which places him in the center of frenetic and often destructive activities. The sick patient needs to be surrounded with peace and love, not the multiple activities so common in most hospitals today. This is not to say that it is not necessary for there to be the multiple analyses, studies, and therapies that are carried out in hospitals. There are varying degrees of illness. In acute illness, many diagnostic studies must be carried out and many activities be concentrated upon the patient. However, as soon as it is possible, it is of utmost importance that the patient be removed from the busy hospital into situations where a more normal and healthful atmosphere can surround him. If this atmosphere can be Christian, with an emphasis on the Medicine of the Whole Person, recovery on all levels of the being will be found to be more rapid than usual. Such an experiment has indeed been carried out in the Medford hospital, and, as a result of almost two years study of this type of medicine, one can conclude that such medical and nursing practice in enlightened hospitals for the terminally and critically ill can be recommended to American medicine and nursing today.

It is important that as a result of the studies carried out in this experiment, American medicine and nursing come to the realization that the nursing home or convalescent hospital image must be changed. In the medicine of the future, it is postulated that there will be an increasing amount of truly acute care carried out in the large hospital situations. Just as there are now postanesthesia recovery rooms and intensive-care units, gradually as the pattern emerges there will be areas in hospitals for the care of patients with acute cardiac conditions such as myocardial infarcts (heart attacks), acute cerebrovascular accidents, pulmonary emboli, and acute renal problems such as those patients who require dialysis and other forms of acute medical care. As soon as the patient is able to be moved out of the situation where acute care is needed, he then can be placed in a situation which is more normal and more like the home situation. There are successful hospitals which have been constructed with this attitude in mind. The nursing home which altogether too often is a place where senile patients are institutionalized to await death, is a relic of the age of neglect of elderly and dying patients. Such facilities should be entirely eliminated from the American medical scene. With the establishment of government programs for medical care of the elderly, many physicians sincerely hope that excellent medical care can be given to all patients no matter what their age or how debilitated, or senile, or chronic they may be. The experiment at the Medford hospital pointed out that such patients can improve tremendously when they are treated as human beings, particularly from the standpoint of Christian care and concern. Such experiments need to be carried out in other situations as a new and enlightened type of care of the elderly, the senile, and the terminally ill appears in American medicine and nursing today, aided by government programs.

One of the rarely considered aspects of medical and nursing care is that aspect of the patient himself. Too often our evaluation of the patient is a statistical one; that is to say: how many days he has been in the hospital, how much of a certain medication he has been given, what his response has been, et cetera. Many times it is a matter of what kind of an operation has been done, whether or not there has been a recurrence of the problem, and how long it has been before the recurrence became apparent. There is a continuing need for there to be an analysis of the response of the patient to the care he receives in the hospital. There also should be more thorough evaluation of the patient's attitude and reaction to medication. Simply because medication can be prescribed and given, does not mean that such medication is always good or carries with it the possibility of ultimate benefit. A letter in *The Lancet* (February 12, 1966) entitled, "What the Patient Felt" has to do with the patient's evaluation of his hospital and medical care during a time when he had a nervous breakdown. Some of the following remarks made by the patient are of interest.

After my nervous breakdown, I was in the hospital for several weeks and I was treated with electric shock and drugs. I don't know whether I am supposed to, but I remember almost every detail and experience.

I was chiefly struck by the godlike detachment of the hospital psychiatrists. To be fair, this varied from man to man, but I got the impression that by and large they thought they could cure anything with drugs and shock, in much the same way as a mechanic tackles engine repair. The atmosphere of the place was such that once I began to recover, I tried to get out as quickly as possible even though I was conscious of not being myself. . . .On the effect of the drugs I was given, I am more sure of my ground. The worst part of the experience was when I began to recover. I could neither read nor follow the television. Occupational therapy needed a tremendous effort—not the actual work, but to take an interest in it. On the other hand, just sitting doing nothing brought no relief. The days dragged terribly. The drugs were apparently tranquilizers, but I certainly did not feel tranquil in the sense of being at peace with the world. It was a sort of a frustration, but what it was I wanted to do, I do not know.

Eventually I found that the best thing was to be doing something which needed absolutely no mental effort. I got into a ritual which seemed to help. I voluntarily mopped the washrooms every morning, polishing the taps, and so forth. I made a point of washing and drying the cutlery. I went for frequent walks. We were supposed to stay in the grounds, but I got several miles away at times. I became quite fond of certain walks on the moors. Looking out for certain objects seemed to engage my attention without requiring effort.

When I was discharged, I still had this terrible feeling. Quite how the doctors decide you are "cured" is a mystery to me. It seems to depend on how many electric shocks you have had. How they decide the particular number of shocks is also a mystery. It seems an arbitrary, ritualistic system to me. Once a week the head doctor came around, an occasion of some importance in the hospital life. Since I wanted to get out quickly, I never answered anything but "fine" when asked how I felt. This was my only direct contact with the medical staff.

From the time I went into the hospital I had been taking some sixteen pills a day. After six weeks at home I suddenly decided that I would stop taking the pills and see what happened. I had a few rough nights, but there was an immediate improvement. I felt more like my old self. Within a week I could read for pleasure. I could just jog along as of old without having to force myself into taking an interest in life. Perhaps this feeling was some peculiar reaction to the drug not experienced by others, but I do not think so. . . .

I hope you don't feel I am making a specific complaint against the hospital. I was in a very bad way and I am grateful to the people who looked after me. It cannot be an easy job. But I feel that I have had to drag myself back into normal life in a way that would not have been necessary if there had been more sympathetic contact with the doctors and less blind faith in drugs and shock.

I do not suppose many psychiatrists have had breakdowns. A patient is not likely to connect his lack of concentration with the drug until he stops taking it.

All in all, I am doubtful whether these drugs are really understood. Certainly a drugged patient behaves very quietly and appears very calm, but in my experience the mental torment is worse than at the height of the delirium. Then your thoughts race, but you are only half-aware that you are ill. Later, you are fully conscious of your illness but can do nothing about it. You have no thoughts; you lead a sort of suspended, frustration existence. The only reason you are quiet is because you don't know what the devil to do with yourself. Some sign from the doctors that they understand how you feel would be a great help. As it is it seems that they have no idea—and if so, how can they really know what they are treating? No doubt many of these impressions were affected by my illness and were illogical. Nonetheless, it is how I felt which matters.

Were patients more often to relate their experiences in hospitals and with doctors and nurses and were the medical and nursing professions to take cognizance of such writings, there would be an improvement in patient care in general; however, we tend to live in a state of detachment from the patient and from the hospital situation. It is necessary for the doctor and the nurse to look more thoroughly at the hospital itself, not just at the laboratory or its operating room, or delivery room, or intensive-care unit, but at the hospital rooms and corridors and the general aspect of the place in which our patients must live. Were we to do this, we would see that such an experiment as was carried out in Medford indeed was one which bears repetition on the scale of larger institutions.

We who profess and call ourselves Christians must see that there should be no difference whatsoever between Christian care and medical and nursing care in general. Certainly, American medicine as it exists at present is an outgrowth of Christian concern for people. Many of our hospitals were established by Christian denominational groups. Somehow, however, we have removed God and Jesus Christ from our consideration. We have become atheistic without realizing it. As long as we practice medicine and nursing without the consideration of God and with no mention of Him, we are basically atheistic whether we choose to actually define ourselves so or not.

American medicine today, by and large, is perhaps as atheistic as was Soviet medicine. The only difference is that Communists realize and profess their atheism, and we have developed our atheism by secondary intention. Such medicine and nursing practice is sterile and not considerate of the deeper aspects of the life of the patient wherein lies not only his true inner spirit and psychological being, but also the key to his recovery and his wholeness while he is in the hospital and especially when he is discharged for care as an outpatient and at home. The few cases cited in the hospital experiment in Medford can serve only as a guide to a more enlightened medical and nursing practice of the future.

It is appropriate in American medicine that now, when great strides are being taken in care of the elderly, many of them chronically and terminally ill, for the Medicine of the Whole Person to be the rule rather than the exception of future practice.

In considering the patient and his reaction to hospitalization and illness in general, there is needed a Patient's Bill of Rights such as follows:

1. The patient has the right to know that he will receive the highest and best nursing and medical care available in order to achieve care and consideration of his spirit, soul, and body.

2. He needs to know that his nursing and medical professionals who care for him are qualified through education, experience, and character to carry out the services for which they are responsible.

3. The patient needs to know that the medical and nursing personnel caring for him will be sensitive to his feelings and responsive to his total need as a person.

4. That within limits determined by his physician, the patient and his family will be taught about the illness besetting the patient, so that he can help himself and his family can understand and help him after his discharge from the hospital.

5. That plans will be made with him and his family, or, if necessary, for him, so that continuing care be available to him throughout the entire period of his need.

6. That adequate records be kept and that confidence be maintained concerning the character of his illness.

7. That a healthful environment be around him in the hospital—an environment which conveys an atmosphere itself conducive to healing.

8. That while he is being treated in mind and body, his spiritual needs also be considered and that if he should be facing death, he may have the opportunity to accept Jesus Christ as his Savior through the combined efforts of the doctor, nurse, and minister.

9. That though he be in coma, or anesthetized, or otherwise without consciousness, he always be treated with love and dignity.

10. That although minority beliefs and practices be always honored and preserved, the right of the Christian to be treated according to the tenets of his Christian belief be also honored, preserved, and practiced.

11. That the patient has the right to know that no matter how critical his situation may be, he never will be denied hope.

A new heart also will I give you, and a new spirit will I put within you: and I will take away the stony heart out of your flesh, and I will give you an heart of flesh. Ezekiel 36:26.

13 - A New Heart

ONTO THE WORLD'S surgical and scientific scene there has recently come the startling phenomenon of the removal of various parts of the body from deceased persons and the reimplantation of organs into patients dying for the lack of healthy organs. The most recent accomplishments have been the transplantation of the heart, lung, liver, and the pancreas. In a book on organ transplantation, the surgeon gives various quotations at the beginning of each chapter. There is one quotation taken from the Holy Bible and it is interesting that it is one of the few quotations of Satan, ". . . Skin for skin, yea, all that a man hath will he give for his life." (Job 2:4). Why this particular quotation was used is difficult to say, except that it does reflect a prophetic truth despite its origin. Man will do anything in order to preserve his temporal life despite the fact that there is God's promise that he will have life eternal through belief in Jesus Christ.

Surgeons will be required in time to come to think more deeply on moral questions than even the theologian or the Christian moralist, since ultimately it is the surgeon who must make the decision to operate and to transplant. It is his hands which do the final act of removing an organ from one individual and transplanting it into another. There are those who would place the physician in the capacity of a technician operating at the bid and call of a board of experts. This concept is loathsome to the surgeon who realizes that his occupation is hardly that of a technician or a carpenter, but is indeed a holy calling given to him by God with all of its awesome responsibility.

A reporter asked a famous American surgeon who has done a number of transplants his opinion of families who refuse permission for the heart to be taken from a loved one to be transplanted into another individual. The doctor said he found such an attitude incomprehensible. He felt that donation of organs should be allowed in every instance. The reporter asked him if the refusal to grant the organ for transplantation were based upon a religious consideration, that is, that the heart is the seat of the soul. The doctor replied that this *had* been the consideration. It was his feeling that *if there is a soul*, it is located in the head and not in the heart.

The purpose of relating this event is simply to point out the fact that now, more than ever, surgeons are having to give consideration to moral and religious questions. Since theirs is the ultimate decision as to whether such operations are to be performed, the education of future physicians and surgeons must not exclude the field of Christian ethics and decision making.

In considering organ transplantation, there is an often-ignored, but all-important, question which must be answered in every instance: Does the potential donor have any chance of survival? Several years ago I was requested to see a young girl who had sustained a cardiac arrest and who had been unconscious for three months. During that time she had been seen by many physicians and specialists; all had concurred: no possibility of recovery. I was asked to see her, not only from the medical standpoint, but also because as a Christian doctor, perhaps I might see her situation from the view point of Christian hope. Entering the hospital room, I was overwhelmed by a picture of complete despair and hopelessness. The child herself was what medicine calls a vegetable. Everyone surrounding her was devoid of hope. Such a patient at such a point could conceivably be considered for organ donation. Most of those surrounding her at the time of my visit were of an opinion that she should be allowed to die. Our decision was to pray and to ask God to heal her. We also made the decision to surround her with love and care, concern and hope. With these as our only *armamentaria*, the child began to respond. Within a few months she was discharged from the hospital.

The decision to carry out organ transplantation must always be done with the knowledge that the person receiving the transplanted organ may die during or shortly after the procedure. The individual who is to be the donor must possess living, healthy organs in order for them to be successfully implanted. Thus the donor must, in a certain sense, be living at the time the organs are removed. By older criteria of death, his respirations have not ceased nor has his heart stopped beating. The brain waves may be flat, but by these new criteria of death, doctors are apt to substitute the findings of a *diagnostic instrument* for clinical diagnosis. In a sense, the donor must die in order for the recipient to have an opportunity to live; therefore there must be great concern and thorough and exhaustive consultation before deciding to allow a person to be a donor. Such operations should only be done at specified centers where there is every facility available for deep moral as well as scientific decisions.

In all instances, the donor is someone who has met with some sort of catastrophe—whether it be an accident or attempted suicide. With the advent of resuscitative methods, such an unfortunate individual may be brought into a hospital emergency service in a state of apparent death. He is then resuscitated and brought back to life so that his heart and vital organs are functioning, excepting perhaps the brain. Were he to live, it is entirely possible that he would live in a state of vegetation for a matter of weeks, months, or years, never regaining consciousness.

There are those instances, however, where people in a state of vegetation have recovered despite every prognostication to the contrary. Thus, the transplant surgeon is faced with a dilemma in which he must obtain the consultation and advice of his fellow physicians and, hopefully, the best minds of men who think upon man not only physically, but spiritually.

It is a Christian principle that the giving up of one's life so that another may live is a manifestation of great love. Jesus Christ said, "Greater love hath no man than this, that a man lay down his life for his friends" (John 15:13). It is a matter of tremendous and soul-searching importance to the individual who has received a transplanted heart as he contemplates the fact that he owes his life not only to the skill and scientific acumen of a number of excellent surgeons, but also that he carries within his being the heart of an individual who died in order that he might live. It is the opinion of such patients that transplant operations are of absolute importance. Certainly their life has depended upon the success of such an operation.

Thus it can be recommended: In order to help to give life to certain productive and critically ill individuals who otherwise face certain death, organ transplantation should be considered. Such operations should never become commonplace. The decisions involved should be based upon the deepest of moral and ethical considerations.

In order to utilize every ethical safeguard, such operations should only be done where the ultimate consideration of all factors is available. The least of these is the technical ability to perform the operation. Surgeons performing such operations should be expert not only in technical phases of operative procedure and aftercare, but they should be more thoroughly grounded than other physicians in the psychological and spiritual considerations of such operative procedures.

The transplant surgeon should have the knowledge, in talking with the family of a prospective donor, that the soul is not located in the heart; nor is it located in the head. The soul is, in fact, the thinking and understanding part of the individual present in all areas of his consciousness. The heart has been called the seat of the understanding (soul). In this instance it does not mean the heart as we understand it but the inner part of one's being.

Thus, in transplanting a heart, there is no transplantation of soul or spirit, but of a physical organ. When the patient has had a severe brain injury—either due to a prolonged lack of oxygen to the brain or a destructive accident which has destroyed the thinking part of the brain—this will be manifested on the electroencephalogram by a characteristic electric pattern. Under these circumstances, the understanding of the individual which includes his will and distinctive attributes of his personality or self are no longer present nor are they retrievable. If one can be certain of this fact, one can with assurance go ahead with the removal of the donor organ or organs if the family allows the organ donation to be done.

The other and perhaps most difficult question is: When does the spirit leave the body? Is the eternal spirit of the individual gone at the moment the soul succumbs? This is doubtless something that we shall never know exactly; however, it is my contention that whatever surgical procedure I am involved in, I shall always consider the patient as spiritually aware of what is happening whether or not he is conscious. If it is impossible to anesthetize the spirit, it is also impossible to destroy the spirit through an accident or through suicide.

It is possible that the third part of man—his spirit—is present in the donor, even at the moment of organ donation. Total physical death ensues at the moment of the organ donation; it is doubtless true that the spirit, if it has not gone to be with God prior to the time, departs at that moment. For the person who is in Christ, this is not a moment to be considered with anxiety or fear, but for the person who is not in Christ, it is indeed a tragic moment. It also would behoove the surgeon who is involved in this moral and ethical problem to be very sure of his ground, spiritually. I would not ever want to make any of these decisions without prayer and the deepest searching for the guidance and direction of God with reference to the proposed procedure. This should be done in every instance. The era of organ transplantation makes it imperative that the surgeon, perhaps more than any other mortal man at this time, must be a man not only of the mind and the soul, but also of the Spirit.

But my God shall supply all your need according to his riches in glory by Christ Jesus. Philippians 4:19.

14 - Prayer

GOD IS NOT LIMITED by the limitations of the minds of men. The Bible promises that God will supply all our needs through Christ Jesus. This does not allow for any limitation or exception. When Jesus Christ lived here on earth He taught men to live in a new dimension of prayer and expectancy. He did not allow anything on the level of the impossible to deter Him or to stop His ministry to the sick. Not even death was able to defeat Him. He demonstrated by raising Lazarus that if the need were for one to be raised from the dead, God can indeed supply that need. With men there are many impossibilities, but ". . . with God all things are possible" (Mark 10:27).

One of the things which characterizes the practice of surgery is the acceptance of the impossibility for some to become well or to totally recover from their illnesses. As one makes his rounds in various hospitals, he cannot help but be aware that many of those whom he sees from day to day—both his patients and others'—are facing imminent death. A hospital is a strange mixture of those who are being preserved for further life and those who are in the acute process of dying. Impossibility lies on every hand. The doctor and the nurse learn to live in this reality.

One night I visited the intensive-care unit of one of our local hospitals. My patient had cancer; and following radical surgery, she was lingering between life and death. A tube was in her throat, and she was unable to talk; however, she wrote a brief note, "Pray for me," and grasped my hand. There in the midst of many others in similar situations, with background sounds of cardiac monitors beeping, occasional desperate cries of patients, and the reassuring replies of nurses, we prayed, asking God to intervene. My patient immediately became calm, and a new courage could be seen to be emanating from her. As I left her and walked down the darkened corridors of the hospital, someone was being taken into the operating room for emergency surgery. Ambulances were bringing other patients into the emergency suite.

I walked by the hospital chapel. No one was there, and its quiet peace summoned me; I slipped inside and lifted up the needs of my patients who were in the hospital that busy night. I also prayed for the physicians and the nurses and asked that God's guiding hand be with them. The chapel seemed like an island of hope in the midst of an ocean of desperation. I breathed a quiet prayer of thanksgiving that someone had had the foresight to see that there was such a place in the hospital for times like this.

After leaving the chapel, I went to visit another patient. Walking down the corridor to see her, I noted on a nearby door a sign "No Ministers Allowed—By Order of the Patient's Doctor." I reflected for a moment as to what such a sign could mean. A nurse, noticing, quietly told me the reason for the sign: The ministers visiting the patient said things such as, "How are you feeling today?" She would reply, "Very well, thank you." Then "Now, you know that I am a minister so you can be honest with me. How do you *really* feel?" In view of the desperate and terminal cancer, everyone reflected discouragement and despair.

Similar conversations and attitudes—all of them more psychological than spiritual—caused the physician to order that no further negativism be allowed. Such statements and philosophy were adding to the patient's burden, rather than lightening it. I heartily concurred with my fellow surgeon's feelings. Those who visit the sick *must* be conveyors of hope. When one has Jesus Christ's life in him, he can see hope even in the most impossible situation. God is the God of the impossible.

If those who claim to be ministers of the Gospel of Jesus Christ cannot encourage, cannot bring faith and hope and healing virtue into sickrooms, they should be forbidden contact with patients. Their place is not to interrogate the patient nor to determine anything concerning the progress of his illness, its physical and psychological attributes.

The minister's primary function is to breathe confidence into the patient's life, to pray for the patient and give whatever ministrations his denomination prescribes. He should leave the patient uplifted and strengthened as a result of his visit. If he does not believe that God exists, if he feels that God is dead or that God does not hear or bring hope to the hopeless, he should not visit the sick. His visits can only be detrimental, even if he does not say a word. A defeatist attitude is lethal to the sick patient whether it emanates from minister, doctor or nurse.

There was a young teenage girl in our community who was dying of a cancerous growth in her arm which had spread into the axilla and the chest wall. Neighbors of the girl—knowing that I was a physician who believed in the healing ministry of

Christ—had asked me if I would visit her to encourage her spiritually, since it was apparent that there was nothing further that could be done for her medically or surgically. I replied that I should be most pleased to visit her if a request for such a visit came from her physician. Shortly thereafter the girl's physician came up to me and asked me, "What do you believe concerning prayer for hopeless patients?" I asked him what he meant. He related that he had been approached by his patient's family and friends regarding having me visit his patient. I explained to him that I had informed them that I would not visit the child unless requested to do so by him. He replied quite indignantly, "I am a Christian and I believe in prayer, and if any doctor is going to pray for my patient, I will do the praying!"

I relate this story only to state that I believe absolutely that this physician was correct. In the ideal situation I do not believe that anyone is any closer to the patient than his physician. The minister or priest may not be as close to the patient as the doctor. The doctor who takes care of his patient physically and psychologically is the logical person to take care of him spiritually.

It is unwise to divide the patient into various parts and areas, since he is a unity and must be cared for always as a whole being. Thus, who can better pray for the patient than his concerned physician? Certainly, a physician rather than a clergyman knows the circumstances of the illness, how serious it may be or its prognosis. Too, a minister's prayers might be misinterpreted by the patient as negative prayers or a form of last rites. The physician should never abandon his patient, even to a minister. The enlightened minister who believes in Christian healing is a wonderful help to patient and physician, but the patient's terminal care spiritually should not be relegated only to him. The doctor or nurse who ignores spiritual involvement with his patient is actually avoiding the issue. Lack of spiritual care and concern are negativistic and destructive to the patient at a time when this aspect of his care becomes all-important and physical and psychological methods become meaningless and fruitless.

Prayer may not necessarily be verbal. Often it is the unspoken prayer which has the greatest result. One time I was discussing prayer with the German psychiatrist, Von Dürckheim. I asked him what his opinion was concerning prayer for patients in the hospital. He replied to me, "There are times when I may have a patient who is possessed of morbid fear. The patient may be afraid to be alone and afraid to be out of my presence. On such occasions I have seen fit from time to time to sit at the bedside all night, holding the patient's hand and reassuring him that everything is alright. This to me is prayer." He then said that occasionally in his practice his patients may require shock therapy. They are brought back following their treatment and placed in their rooms. Von Dürckheim spoke of the importance of the *kind of eyes* they would see when awakening from their treatment. Eyes of love, care, and concern differ from those which are impersonal or irritated and upset. One's eyes speak prayer. His attitude bespeaks prayer. A life speaks prayer—or it does not. A man is either plus or minus spiritually; he cannot be neutral.

I began to think about Christianity as ordinarily practiced, and it occurred to me that Christianity is often a spoken religion. Prayers are those things which are said or read out of a prayer book. Christianity is often conceived as the history detailed in the New Testament, the proclamation that those who believe in Jesus Christ will be saved to life eternal.

There is, however, I am sure, a greater depth and a greater

reality to the life of Jesus Christ who lives within the believer. It cannot be just what is being said or just what is being proclaimed in the pulpit or in the witness at the Christian Men's Club. It must be something that is being *lived*, not in the power of the individual, but in the power of Jesus' Resurrection. Such a *living faith* in the sickroom and in the psychiatric wards is needed in all of those places where the sick person longs not just to *hear* a prayer but to *see* vital, quickening Christianity lived and practiced in the lives of those who care for him in his hour of need.

Were this to be the case there would be no need for signs to be placed on patients' doors saying "No Ministers Allowed". This is a dimension of Christian hope of which the physician and the nurse are perhaps better qualified to evaluate and be a part of than anyone else. They are on the front lines fighting death and disease. The physician, perhaps more than most other mortal men, needs the strengthening power of the Holy Spirit and the virtue of Jesus Christ in his life. Alone he is constantly being sapped of healing virtue. He is a channel of the healing love of God through Jesus Christ, whether he chooses to believe this fact or not. He has the gift of healing which is a gift of God and the Holy Spirit, whether he has ever accepted the precepts of Christianity or not. How much greater his results would be, not only on the temporal but on the eternal scale, if he were to see that he is indeed a co-laborer with God as he goes about his daily endeavors in the healing of the sick. He would then have a constant and ever-increasing supply of compassion, love, and strength in order to meet the myriad needs of the multitudes of sick whom he sees every day. The physician cannot carry all of these burdens alone, but with the power of Christ indwelling, he will find that he has a new strength and is no longer drained of life, joy, and victory, as is so often the case when one attempts to heal the sick, relying only on his own human frailty and in the human efforts of those who surround him—however conscientious and however laudable.

My patient in the intensive-care suite, following prayer, began to get well and soon was discharged from the hospital. Not only was she healed of the immediate problem but God has continued to heal her in all areas of her spirit, soul, and body. This truly is the ultimate purpose of the physician's life and of the Christian's life—those who believe in and trust the Lord Jesus Christ. The Christian must uniquely portray the healing power of Christ; otherwise, he is proclaimer of something other than the Gospel. The Gospel message is a healing message, and not only are doctors and nurses in need of its possession in their own lives, but man in general, in the desperate hour in which we live in the world today, needs the healing Gospel of Jesus as in no other previous time.

Grace and peace be multiplied unto you through the knowledge of God, and of Jesus our Lord, According as his divine power hath given unto us all things that pertain unto life and godliness, through the knowledge of him that hath called us to glory and virtue: Whereby are given unto us exceeding great and precious promises: that by these ye might be partakers of the divine nature, having escaped the corruption that is in the world through lust. 2 Peter 1:2-4.

15 - Death and Dying

THERE IS MUCH THOUGHT being given today to the subject of death and dying. Perhaps this is not unusual, since there has been no time in the recorded annals of man in which so many human beings have been subjected to premature and violent death as in the twentieth century. This is a strange paradox, since civilization has achieved its zenith in many ways, especially in the realm of science and medicine in this century. It could be stated as an inverse proportion: The higher the scientific culture, the greater the incidence of violent death. If we are advancing in our generation scientifically, we must then expect more death and more violence, unless God intervenes. As science and the biologic orientation of life achieve the ascendancy, the spiritual and the cultural orientations of life diminish. God and His Church are replaced by mathematical formulas and scientific rules and practices. New gods are developed, and the people of the world eagerly follow first one temporal deity and then another. One result of this orientation of man toward science rather than toward God has been the new death-and-dying movement.

First it is necessary to consider some of the statements and beliefs of the death-and-dying movement, after which we shall attempt to determine if there is a different point of view which can obtain end results more beneficial and not exclude what Peter defines as the "hope that lies within us" (*see* 1 Peter 3:15). An attempt must be made to identify whether the basic idea of resignation to death, and cooperation with that resignation, is a true Judeo-Christian concept, or whether it is not. If it is not, and if the leaders of the death-and-dying movement have pointed out a great flaw in the care of the terminally ill, there is urgent need for the immediate development of a Christian philosophy of the care of the "medically hopeless" based upon biblical bases. Terminal illness in the Christian sense can be defined as not having Jesus in one's heart.

Before considering the death-and-dying movement, let us briefly consider the semantics of the question. What does it mean to be *terminal*, to have a terminal illness? Terminal is defined as referring to time, particularly pertaining to the end of a period; in this instance, the end of life. Medically it refers to the possession of an illness or a scenario of illnesses from which there is no possibility of recovery. At the termination of the process of whatever sort, death ensues. The process prior to death has been termed *dying*. In order for there to be a study of how to care for the dying patient, we need to determine when the patient is in truth dying. When is the dying patient to be placed in a palliative-care center? When do physician, nurse, and clergyman advise the necessity of stopping life-support systems? When does this process become euthanasia (*eu:* normal; *thanatos*: death)? Is there such a thing as normal death? Does a Christian Die? In the Service of Holy Communion of the Anglican Church, dating back to the sixteenth century, we read, "And we most humble beseech thee, of thy goodness, O Lord, to comfort and succour all those who, *in this transitory life*, are in trouble, sorrow, need, sickness, or any other adversity."

Thus life is seen in the Christian sense as being transitory and bearing with it a terminus from the moment of conception. ". . . For what is your life? It is even a vapour, that appeareth for a little time, and then vanisheth away." (James 4:14). This life is something man cannot will to hold tightly and completely within his own grasp. Jesus has taught us ". . . whosoever will save his life shall lose it: but whosoever will lose his life for my sake, the same shall save it." (Luke 9:24). Thus, in the Christian sense, it is difficult to talk about terminal illness, and even to consider dying with the finality of the writers of death and dying. In this discussion, the term *medically hopeless* will be applied to patients who have disease states in which, at this stage of our lack of enlightenment, we are unable to produce healing through the utilization of medical, scientific means.

The writers in the death-and-dying movement have helped both patients and those who care for them by identifying the fact that modern medicine does not adequately care for or help those who are medically hopeless. With all that has been written and said, the problem is so great that the surface of this consideration has barely been touched. Until the beginning of the twentieth century, much of the concern of those who cared for the sick was the care of the dying. Many medical methods actually eventuated in death. Consider here purging, bleeding, and leeching which were the common methods of medical healing less than one hundred years ago. Since the beginning of our present century, great medical, surgical, and scientific advances have been made. With the advent of antibiotic therapy, countless numbers of lives have been saved which previously would have been lost to bacterial and infectious diseases. Antibiotics, anesthesia, and increased knowledge of physiology and body-and-blood chemistry have made possible tremendous advances in surgery. At the present time, the advances in bio-engineering and immunology open new horizons of medical discovery and treatment.

On the surface, all of this may appear to be good and beneficial. Problems have begun to surface, and as a result, those who have become concerned with death and the process of dying have begun to voice their anxieties. It would seem rather strange that the Church has not had more to say in this regard. It has become apparent that it is possible to prolong bodily function even after it is ascertainable that vital life processes (soul and spirit functions in the body) have greatly diminished or ceased. This is particularly true in patients who have had brain injury, massive strokes, coma, or what has been termed multiple-systems failure. In these instances, imminent death is apparent, and most families and their physicians insist that life under these conditions not be prolonged, particularly when electroencephalographic tracings indicate brain death. Certainly for the Christian whose hope is in God and in eternal life, this decision is not difficult to arrive at. For the person who is not saved and has no hope in Christ, this is a most difficult juncture to arrive at, making it urgent that those who preach, teach, and heal, lead all men to Christ while they are yet able to ask Jesus to forgive and save them.

In other instances, approaching death may not be quite as obvious or as ascertainable, either on the part of the patient or the physician. The prognosis of approaching death can be made through appraising the nature of the disease process, the knowledge of its usual course, and the possible effectiveness of available treatment. There is always the factor of the patient himself, his resistance and, for Christians, the hope of the healing Savior (*see* John 14:13,14).

Those writing and speaking about death and dying have had specific recommendations to set forth regarding dying patients. Their emphasis has been primarily upon death and its probable irreversibility. The basic tenets of the teaching of this movement are as follows (gleaned from writings and conferences):

1. The patient has a right to relief of symptoms.

2. The patient does not have to die in pain and distress.

3. Death is a part of life.

4. The physician must talk to the patient regarding his approaching death.

5. The time comes when usual methods of treatment and medications must be stopped.

6. Ordinary medicine and the "medicine of death and dying" are systems in conflict.

a) Ordinary medicine wants to keep trying; to try something else; to not face the fact of approaching death; to use every kind of treatment and device until the bitter end.

b) Death-and-dying medicine has been defined as high-person, low-technology care.

7. The aim is growth in maturity.

8. It is not just the patient who is dying. Consider his family and loved ones.

9. Death is seen by the doctor as failure. We do not want to face our failures. Thus we may neglect our dying patient.

10. In every instance, it must be determined whether an illness is remedial or deteriorating toward death.

11. There is never such a thing as "nothing can be done."

12. In *On Death and Dying*, Dr. Elizabeth Kubler-Ross describes the various stages the patient may go through as he approaches his death. The stage of denial is usually first, followed by a stormy period of anger, when the patient may become insulting, irritating, and complaining. This should not be taken personally by the doctor or the nurse, and it is certainly not a time to avoid the patient. The third stage might be one of bargaining (usually with God) for an extension of time. In the fourth stage, there occurs grief and the facing of future losses and the beginning of preparation for the eventual death. Acceptance is usually the last stage, as all that has to be said is said and all the unfinished business has been addressed.

13. Concentration must be made upon the quality of remaining life in all efforts extended toward the patient.

As one considers the above, very little fault can be found concerning the principles of the death-and-dying movement; however, with deeper reflection, there are seen to be several deficiencies. Most important is the failure to consider hope and the lack of emphasis upon life and living. As with all modern medical approaches, there is little spiritual consideration. *Is* it a laudable objective to advocate the principle of death with dignity and without pain or distress, and not to consider the place of prayer and peace with God? Is pain always a bad thing? May not suffering lead a patient to the point of making his peace with God? Are narcotics the only means of pain relief? Has anyone ever considered prayer as a method of achieving peace and relief from fear and pain?

Regarding death, what did Jesus mean when He said "And whosoever liveth and believeth in me shall never die . . ."? (John 11:26.) In the Gospels, whenever Jesus encountered death or those who were dying, He reflected the fact that He *is* the Resurrection and the Life, and demonstrated that fact by giving life and healing. He also instructed His disciples and the other seventy (*see* Luke 9 and 10) to go out and preach and heal the sick. Jesus commanded His disciples to raise the dead. It is apparent that the Gospel message is not one of resignation to illness and death. Jesus said, ". . . I am come that they might have life, and that they might have it more abundantly." (John 10:10).

When we are born again, when we posses Jesus, we have more than just a pleasant philosophy of life. We are possessors of God Himself. We have His creation power. Paul tells us that our potential is to be persons filled with all of the fullness of God. This is what we carry to our patients—to the sick, the hopeless, the anxious, the suffering, and the dying. We truly have a power to live by and a dynamic to share. The Christian faith is a great and tremendous power. It is life itself, in contrast to death. We then are conveyors of life—eternal life, Resurrection power—

when we are filled with the Holy Spirit. We may remember the inspiring hymn of W. Howard Doane and Fanny J. Crosby of a century ago:

> Down in the human heart, crushed by the tempter,
> Feelings lie buried that grace can restore;
> Touched by a loving hand, wakened by kindness,
> Chords that were broken will vibrate once more.
> Rescue the perishing, Care for the dying;
> Jesus is merciful, Jesus will save.

Paul, in 2 Corinthians 4:3, has written, "But if our gospel be hid, it is hid to them that are lost." The *Amplified Bible* says it is hid to those who are "perishing." As Christians, our primary responsibility is to live Jesus Christ. In living and proclaiming Him, we rescue the perishing. As Christians who care for the sick and the dying, our primary responsibility is to care for the dying.

What does it mean to care for the dying? Consider Luke 10:25-29, where Jesus, in talking with a certain lawyer, had been asked:

> ". . . what shall I do to inherit eternal life? He said unto him, What is written in the law? how readest thou? And he answering said, Thou shalt love the Lord thy God with all thy heart, and with all thy soul, and with all thy strength, and with all thy mind; and thy neighbour as thyself. And he said unto him, Thou hast answered right: this do, and thou shalt live. But he, willing to justify himself, said unto Jesus, And who is my neighbour?"

Jesus then related the parable of the man from Jerusalem who went to Jericho and fell among thieves. A case of trauma—a person dying (half-dead)—who was neglected by a priest and a Levite (one of the Levitical priesthood), but ministered to by a Samaritan who had compassion on him, went to him, bound up his wounds and, pouring in oil and wine, set him on his own beast and brought him to an inn. The Samaritan paid for his care and obligated himself for future cost.

"Which now of these three, thinkest thou, was neighbour unto him that fell among the thieves? And he said, He that shewed mercy on him. Then said Jesus unto him, Go, and do thou likewise." (Luke 10:36, 37). This is what it means to care for the dying.

Who are the dying? "For the living know that they shall die. . ." (Ecclesiastes 9:5). "But of the tree of the knowledge of good and evil, thou shalt not eat of it: for in the day that thou eatest thereof thou shalt surely die." (Genesis 2:17). "For the wages of sin is death; but the gift of God is eternal life through Jesus Christ our Lord." (Romans 6:23). In our natural Adamic state, we are all dying. "For as in Adam all die, even so in Christ shall all be made alive." (1 Corinthians 15:22).

We are all terminal (in the Adamic sense). The cancer patient who has metastatic disease knows, somewhat more realistically than we, the time of his approaching death. Thus the dying patient is me—myself. He also could be Jesus. ". . .Inasmuch as ye have done it unto one of the least of these my brethren, ye have done it unto me" (Matthew 25:40).

"For I was an hungred, and ye gave me meat: I was thirsty, and ye gave me drink: I was a stranger, and ye took me in: Naked, and ye clothed me: I was sick, and ye visited me: I was in prison, and ye came unto me." (Matthew 25:35, 36).

The dying patients are on every side. Some are more obvious than others. The most urgent need in the consideration of the dying patient is for there to be general understanding of the spiritual nature of man and how, as doctors and nurses and ministers and aides, we can help those who are approaching death. We need to realize that man is not just mind and body—not just psychosomatic—but he is also spirit (*see* 1 Thessalonians 5:23 and Hebrews 4:12).

In all phases of illness, the patient requires ministry on all three levels of his being, but this is especially true for the dying patient. To ignore the spirit is to treat that patient negatively from the spiritual point of view. As the psychosomatic decreases, the spiritual increases in importance. The closer the patient comes to death, the more important the spiritual becomes.

The types of spiritual patient care are compassion, having vital contact with the patient, and taking care of him. The Scriptures show that we must teach and heal, bestow peace, and use the laying on of hands and anointing.

There is a difference between taking care of a psychosomatic (unsaved) or a born-again patient. The patient who is born again, and knows it, is not a patient who views death with fear. He rarely, in my experience, goes through the Elizabeth Kubler-Ross stages of death and dying. Dr. Paul Tournier's doctor friend (a Christian) said that he desired no narcotics as his death approached. He stated, "I will not allow anyone to steal my death from me."

I am convinced that fear and apprehension cause pain to increase. Many of my postoperative patients require no postoperative narcotic medications. Narcotics and sedatives are prescribed, but are usually not asked for.

There is an urgent need of empowerment of the Holy Spirit in those who care for the dying (and all patients). A Spirit-filled medical priesthood is needed, so that the area of the spirit in patient care may be considered intensively—to the same or greater degree to which we study and treat the mind and body.

The physician and nurse are taking care of the spirit, mind, and body in all patients. If one ignores the mind, he is treating the patient negatively psychologically. If he ignores the spirit, he is treating the patient negatively insofar as the spirit is concerned.

Finally, let us remember that on the cross Jesus defeated sin, the devil, sickness, and death (*see* 1 Peter 2:24). Let us begin to live and work in His accomplished victory.

Sick patients not only ask for those who care for them to be well trained, and scientific, but they also ask for caring, understanding, loving, happy human beings who will not abandon them and will give them Christlike care. As with the disciples, we have peace which we can bestow. We also can possess the gifts of the Holy Spirit, which include gifts of healings and miracles. "And beside this, giving all diligence, add to your faith virtue; and to virtue knowledge; And to knowledge temperance; and to temperance patience; and to patience godliness; And to godliness brotherly kindness; and to brotherly kindness charity." (2 Peter 1:5-7).

This final admonishment is to both physician and patient. All mankind needs healing today, and only through Jesus Christ and His Holy Spirit can man become whole. Medicine, psychiatry, and nursing have largely forgotten the Lord and Giver of life, but a new wave of God's love is creating a new medicine and a new beautiful hope.

Now the mind of the flesh [which is sense and reason without the Holy Spirit] is death . . . But the mind of the [Holy] Spirit is life and . . . peace . . . Romans 8:6 (AMP)

It is the Spirit Who gives life [He is the Life-giver]; the flesh conveys no benefit whatever . . . John 6:63 (AMP)

. . . may your spirit and soul and body be preserved sound and complete [and found] blameless at the coming of our Lord Jesus Christ. . . I Thessalonians 5:23 (AMP)

16 - Logo-Psychosomatic Medicine

WHEN EPHRAIM MCDOWELL, a Kentucky physician and surgeon, performed the first laparotomy in 1809 he prayed: "Almighty God, be with me, I humbly beseech Thee, in this attendance in Thy holy hour; give me becoming awe of Thy presence, and grant me Thy direction and aid. I beseech Thee that in confessing I may be humble and truly penitent in prayer, serious and devout in praises, grateful and sincere, and in hearing Thy Word attentive and willing and desirous to be instructed. Direct me, Oh God, in performing this operation for I am but an instrument in Thy hands and am but Thy servant, and if it is Thy will, Oh spare this poor afflicted woman! Oh give me true faith in the atonement of Thy Son, Jesus Christ, or a love sufficient to procure Thy favor and blessing that worshipping Thee in spirit and in truth my services may be accepted through His all sufficient merit. Amen."

Ephraim McDowell typifies the Christian approach to the patient. The Christian discipline is the absolute foundation of man becoming whole. Christianity is the synthesis of Old Testament and New Testament truth showing man his true identity and the reason for his existence. Christ as Melchizedek, the Angel of the Lord or Messiah, always brings healing. This is seen not only in the life of Moses in the healing of Miriam of leprosy, but also in the healings performed through Elijah and Elisha and in the healing of Hezekiah. In the Old Testament a healing God bestows loving wholeness upon those who love Him. The Ten Commandments list the laws which lead to wholeness and length of days in this life.

In the New Testament there are many healings by Jesus of Nazareth and His disciples as well as those who followed the disciples. Jesus instructed His disciples to go out and to proclaim that God's kingdom was present and demonstrate that fact by healing the sick. In the Gospel of Luke, the physician, Jesus gave His disciples authority "over all devils and to cure diseases." The disciples went about "healing every where." Jesus Himself is never powerless insofar as the healing of the sick is concerned. The multitudes pressed upon Him and He healed them all. St. Paul and St. Peter are both credited with the healing of many people. The power of the Holy Spirit in St. Peter was so great that his shadow could heal. It is recorded that cloths taken from Paul healed those people to whom they were applied. God's Word tells of this miraculous power being present in the totally committed Christian who is filled with God's Spirit. The reason why these things do not happen today is because man has lost his ability to believe totally in God.

In the early Christian era such writers as Tertullian and Cyprian, as well as Origen, Irenaeus, Clement of Alexandria, Hippolytus, Polycarp, Clement of Rome, Ignatius and many others wrote about the power of the Christian life to conquer death and disease. It was not just a Christian discipline but also was a part of Judaism going on into the Middle Ages to the time of Maimonides who wrote about the healing power of God in man's life, especially those who live a holy and consecrated life.

Christianity is erroneously blamed for the time when scientific advance did not continue and when superstition and ignorance reigned during the Dark Ages. However, scholarship and what little was known concerning anatomy and the treatment of illness was preserved in the monasteries of Europe. As man emerged into the scientific era, through the endeavors of such people as Ephraim McDowell and Beaumont, as well as William Harvey, Koch, Pasteur and many others, scientific medicine gradually became an entity which had connections with the church. However, contacts with the church became more and more tenuous. With the advance of pathology and the German Virchow school of thought in the early 20th century, there was a gradual increase in adherence to pure science without consideration of the spiritual aspect of man.

Sigmund Freud and his followers began the attempt to understand the mental aspect of man and the psychiatric difficulties consequent to his relationship to those about him. There emerged a type of medical practice, through the concepts of

Flanders Dunbar in the early 1930's called psychosomatic medicine. Medical practice today is considered to be antiquated unless man is considered as a psychosomatic entity. However, there has been, in recent years, a greater and greater degree of specialization as the knowledge explosion continues. Man is really not considered psychosomatically but is fragmented to the point where it is the rare physician who is able to put him back together physically or psychosomatically. In the 1800's men were closer to God. If they were physicians, they thought of God in relation to themselves and their patients.

We have seen a gradual departure from this type of thinking although there have been such men as Howard Kelly, the great professor of gynecology at Johns Hopkins, who were men of prayer and vocal in their belief in God and His place in the healing of the sick.

Inspirational Philosophies

Austria produced Victor Frankl. He was a product of the universities of the Hitlerian era and developed his philosophy as a result of experiences in concentration camps. Alexis Carrel, A Roman Catholic born in France, was a man whose medical philosophy was deeply affected by a trip to Lourdes, detailed in a little book called "Voyage to Lourdes." After Carrel came to the Flexner Institute in New York City, he became a pioneer researcher in vascular surgery. More important, he was a person who looked very deeply into man. In *Man, the Unknown* he searches into the meaning of life.

Dr. Paul Tournier saw that many of his patients had problems beyond those which could be handled by the writing of prescriptions or by surgery. Practicing in Switzerland he worked with the Red Cross and became a member of the Oxford Movement. His life became oriented toward God and toward the Bible and from his thought and his experiences he developed "The Medicine of the Person." Physicians of all disciplines began to listen to Tournier and attend his conferences in Europe. Dr. Tournier taught that the physician must look deeper into the life of his patient. In order to truly be able to understand man, according to Tournier, doctors must have an experience with God and must point the patient to his personal potential of having an experience with God through Jesus Christ. Tournier's many writings have been an inspiration to the physicians of America who see the danger of increasing scientism and materialism in the practice of medicine and the lack of a true orientation toward the individual who is ill. Both Alexis Carrel and Paul Tournier have joined Victor Frankl in requesting that man become again concerned with himself as a total human being, and with his orientation to God in order to be able to live in the future.

Alexis Carrel in *Man, the Unknown* states that "No one understands that the structural, functional and mental quality of each individual has to be improved. The health of the intelligence and of the affective sense, moral discipline and spiritual development are just as necessary as the health of the body and prevention of infectious diseases. . .Man must now turn his attention to himself and to the cause of his moral and intellectual disability. What is the good of increasing the comfort, the luxury, the beauty, the size and the complications of our civilization if our weakness prevents us from guiding it to our best advantage?...There is not a shadow of a doubt that mechanical, physical and chemical sciences are incapable of giving us intelligence, moral discipline, health, nervous equilibrium, security and peace. . .We must leave the physical and physiological in order to follow the mental and the spiritual."

Dr. Carrel also states, "The new science must progress by a double effort of analysis and synthesis toward a conception of the human individual at once sufficiently complete and sufficiently simple to serve as the basis of our action." We continue to divide man up and we fail to synthesize him into a total whole organism.

With reference to the Church, Dr. Carrel says, "Ministers have rationalized religion. They have destroyed its mystical basis but they do not succeed in attracting modern men." It would be well if, in the crises in the homes and the medical schools of America, the modern physician would go back and read again the writings of Carrel and develop a medicine of wholeness and begin to be healthy and whole himself.

Victor Frankl states in his book, *The Doctor and the Soul*: "Man lives in three dimensions: The somatic, the mental and the spiritual. The spiritual dimension cannot be ignored for it is what makes us human." Proper diagnosis can be made only by someone who can see the spiritual side of man. Psychotherapy alone is insufficient. Frankl advocates a "medical ministry" which would not in any way attempt to substitute for the minister or priest. He states that psychotherapy aims to heal the soul and is essentially different from religion which concerns itself with saving the soul. "Religion provides a man with a spiritual anchor . . . Although the psychotherapist is not concerned with helping his patient achieve a capacity for faith, in certain felicitous cases, the patient regains his capacity for faith. Such a result can never be the end of psychotherapy from the start and a doctor will have to always beware of forcing his philosophy upon the patient . . . The therapist must be careful to see that the patient does not shift his responsibilities onto the doctor." Frankl states that the ultimate consequences of the theory that man is nothing but the product of heredity and environment, has produced, in its most terrible form, the gas chambers of Auschwitz. Of course this same sort of philosophy has allowed a creeping in of the materialistic point of view so that the Auschwitz philosophy has permeated the minds of the majority of our people. This is particularly true in medicine where there has been no consideration of the spiritual aspect of man. Thus Kevorkian and Derek Humphrey have been produced.

In the fact that we have been able to rationalize abortion and human experimentation, we see ourselves gradually falling into the kind of viewpoint which in Germany under Hitler allowed gas chambers to destroy life. Similar places of extermination existed in the Soviet Union according to the writings of Solzhenitsyn.

Victor Frankl has stated that there is a blank area in the science of psychotherapy which awaits filling. Psychotherapy was born when the attempt was first made to look behind physical symptoms for psychic causes to discover psychogenesis. Now, "further steps must be taken to look beyond psychogenesis past the affect dynamics of neurosis in order to see distress of the human spirit. The physician and the patient must look into the meaning of life." "We do not strike to the heart to find out what is truly wrong with man any more than a doctor who, completely eschewing any psychotherapeutic approach contents himself with physical treatment or the prescription of medicaments. . .How many rivers of tincture of valerian have flowed for this reason—

just so the doctor would seem to be doing something? How wise, by contrast, is the classic dictum, 'physic the mind and the body will need no physics.' The point is that all such medical approaches in the face of philosophical conflicts amount to working at cross purposes with the patient under pretense of being scientific." Dr. Frankl would advocate the development of a medicine of the soul and spirit. He would call it "medical ministry."

Writings of Evans

Griffith Evans, writing in the 1950's in England, was a surgeon who felt that man was suffering because medical science did not allow man to think in the terms of who he truly is and what his ultimate objective in life should be. He felt that medicine was still in the Newtonian Era and had not begun to think in Einsteinian terms. He accused medicine of having an atomic viewpoint rather than thinking upon man in terms of wave mechanics and the true nature of energy systems. Dr. Evans foresaw a phenomenon of our own present age where, despite the field of organ transplantation and our understanding of gene replication and genetic manipulation, science would be calling for more scientific discoveries and set its hopes on "materialistic horses and chariots." However, he did see that in England in the 1950's and early 1960's some physicians turned to the paranormal and psychic areas of healing and this was symptomatic of man searching for other modes of therapy. He saw in this a danger that man might turn away from true spiritual search and go into the study of the psyche rather than to see the person as a spiritual creation of a spiritual God. Man is not just mind and body but also spirit.

The writings of Griffith Evans are complex, mathematical and most interesting. He envisages the medicine of the future, great in terms of science and also great in knowledge of how man is healed by the power of God—a scientific and spiritual medicine where doctors who are oriented toward God through prayer and oriented toward their patients through love, produce the healing of disease and ultimate wholeness.

Dr. Evans states, "The credibility of the Bible as a divinely inspired and intuitively perceived system of thought also emerges. Insofar as universal human urges are divinely inspired and truly evolutionary, they are irresistible. . .Woe betide the imposed system of academic medicine which disregards Vis Mediatrix Naturae and stand for the false doctrine that civilized substitution therapy is preferable to natural homeostasis." There are natural tendencies within the human body which is always attempting to heal itself. We must learn how to work along with these forces instead of counteracting them through the use of surgery, pharmacology, chemotherapy, and radiation. Dr. Evans implies that we are in modern medicine working at the end results of abnormalities which are termed disease and do not understand the development of disease and the way that the body heals itself and how to cooperate with the natural forces. This can only be understood as we begin to understand the Bible and to understand man intuitively as well as experimentally. He states, "The abandonment of God the Creator as a unifying and restoring principle leaves man at the mercy of incomplete theories and laws of chance." Jung retained the intuitive belief in God and insisted that mental balance could only be restored by reunion with Him who guided its creation and development. The same pattern emerges in every stage of scientific and religious study—a single objective truth and two opposing interpretations: Humanist: based on reason and induction; Theist: based on intuition, deduction and divine guidance. We are in this same position today. Great advances are being made in medicine and surgery but our society is not any healthier. Soulish methodologies excluding spirituality in large measure have failed.

The surgeon who contents himself with taking out an occasional appendix and gall bladder and ignores the illness of society is an incomplete individual. The thinking physician cannot be complacent in the world of today. The great advances in science and the development of material comforts has little meaning to the person who sees the mental and spiritual anguish of the world.

Thus, man must evolve a "new medicine."

Dr. Flanders Dunbar, 40 years ago developed psychosomatic medicine. Supposedly today thinking physicians use psychosomatic medicine in the understanding and therapy of all of their patients. However, specialization is on the increase and few physicians are interested in general practice and the treating of the whole person. Basically, medicine across the world has never been less psychosomatically oriented and there is little or no consideration of the spiritual and eternal aspect of man.

From the writings of the physicians mentioned earlier it is apparent that a great new medicine must be evolved. Dr. Frankl conceived logo-therapy as a new type of psychotherapy. However, the spirit is not an extension of the mind. It is the godly or potentially godly aspect of man. Jesus of Nazareth told Nicodemus it was necessary that he be born of the Spirit. The writings of Watchman Nee of China during the 1920's and 30's are most interesting in this regard. He has written extensively on the necessity of natural man to become spiritual.

Medicine today is a natural medicine practiced by men who have basically ignored the spiritual aspect, not only of their patients but also of themselves. The entire area of the medicine of the Spirit, or what we have termed logo-psychosomatic medicine, appears as a wide-open, uninvestigated and even an unthought of field. There are many illnesses which are conceived of as being psychiatric which are basically spiritual in their origin. There are many illnesses which are a combination of the spiritual as well as psychiatric.

We have found that disorders and anomalies of spiritual development may result in illness in the psychosoma, being an end result of an abnormality which begins in the soul and the spirit. Writers in recent years in psychiatric journals have shown that patients with malignancies often have deep lying psychiatric problems. It is entirely possible that these problems are not only psychiatric but psychospiritual. I have seen the development of cancer of the breast in patients who have deep resentments present in their lives, and have seen the amelioration of the disease process when these deep psychospiritual lethal attributes of the subconscious mind can be dealt with spiritually. One of the great problems in modern medicine is the hiatus between the physician and the psychiatrist and between the doctor and God. Perhaps the family practitioner has the greatest chance of being the doctor of the new medicine. This cannot automatically come about on the basis of suddenly making the decision to become a logo-psychosomatic physician. To use the terms of Jesus, it is necessary for a physician who would adopt the new medicine to become born again, to be born of the Spirit. He will then seek spiritual fellowship with like-minded physicians and nurses. He will see his patients as those who also need to be born of the spirit in order to be totally healed.

The Necessary Transformation

Transformation has been thought of as the function of the church. There has been a wide separation between the minister and the physician. The physician who has become a Christian or a member of the Orthodox Judaic Church has been loathe to inject his thoughts or feelings into his relationship with his patient. It is necessary that the patient come to a decision in his own life as to whether or not he would become spiritual through the personal acceptance of Jesus Christ as Savior. The avenues of transcendental meditation and other new age "religious" systems of the world allude to such a transformation but usually the requirement is the development of an asceticism or a type of metaphysical belief apart from Christ. In the Christian life, spirituality, through the person being born of the Holy Spirit, can be achieved in the midst of the throng and the press of life by simply asking God that one may receive His Holy Spirit. Initially it is necessary for man to accept the life and the Person of Christ. He must ask that the Christ-life principle enter into his life so that he may no longer be simply a man of body and mind but also of Spirit. This is a point of view which is promulgated in the gospels of Jesus Christ and the epistles of the New Testament. If one would desire to investigate this type of transformation, the Holy Bible is the primary book of reference.

In born again man who through the indwelling Christ is developing spirituality, an entirely new area of investigation is opened up for those who are studying the healing of the sick.

Physicians who have been mentioned earlier are men who understood this concept. The realm of the Spirit is not to be confused with spiritualism or occultism despite their erroneous use of the term "spirituality." The psychic or soul realm is a most powerful area of man's being and has tremendous potential for good and evil. However, it is in this mental realm that all of the mind cults including religious science, spiritualism, voodooism and Satanism are found. It is not my purpose to condemn psychic healing or psychic investigation but to advocate by contrast the true in comparison to the incomplete. I believe that psychiatrists and psychologists must understand the counter-balance of the life of the Spirit in order to be able to safely and successfully help patients who have illnesses in the realm of the psyche.

Physicians who are investigating spirituality do not have to abandon traditional medicine in order to become logo-psychosomatic practitioners. The doctor using logo-psychosomatic medical principles finds that if he is an internist, he continues to practice traditional internal medicine but he does so in a much more compassionate and empathetic manner. He has a deeper consciousness of the person of his patient. If he is a surgeon, he is interested in the entire person of the patient and is reverent even during times of the patient's unconsciousness in the post-anesthesia recovery unit or in the operating room. The physician who is working in neurology and dealing with patients who are comatose gives greater reverence than is ordinarily the case and such terms as the patient being a "vegetable" are abandoned since the patient's spirit is always aware.

Logo-psychosomatic medicine is a new medicine for the future which has as its central theme a greater orientation of both doctor and patient toward God through Jesus Christ and through the Holy Spirit. It begins with the physician who must be born of the Spirit. This is a type of medical practice that cannot be administered empirically or without involvement of the physician himself in the deepest areas of his own being. It is a challenging but a most rewarding area of endeavor, not only from the standpoint of determining the etiology of disease but of the treatment and the prevention of illness. Much needs to be done in the realm of investigation. Much needs to be done in the understanding of logo-therapy. Since a man has a spirit, there must be a therapy of spiritual disorders just as a man who has a psyche at times develops psychiatric disorders which have their own psychiatric treatments. Those things which are physical have their physical treatments. However, Flanders Dunbar has shown us that none of these areas exist in airtight compartments. Therefore, psychiatric illness has its spiritual aspects as well as its physical, and spiritual illness has its psychiatric and physical attributes. An expansion is thus needed in man's thinking in all these areas. We must stop concerning ourselves with all of the multiple things that exist peripheral to man and now begin to understand man, the unknown, who is actually man, the creation of God. Man can never be truly understood or treated totally without including God and His Holy Spirit in the therapeutic regimen.